DATE DUE

BREAST CANCER

BREAST CANCER

*A Psychological
Treatment Manual*

Sandra Haber, PhD (Editor)
Catherine Acuff, PhD
Lauren Ayers, PhD
Esther Lerman Freeman, PsyD
Carol Goodheart, EdD
Christine C. Kieffer, PhD
Louise B. Lubin, PhD
Susan G. Mikesell, PhD
Michele Siegel, PhD
Barbara R. Wainrib, EdD

Springer Publishing Company

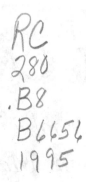

Cover design by Tom Yabut

Springer Publishing Company, Inc.
536 Broadway
New York, NY 10012

95 96 97 98 99 / 5 4 3 2 1

Library of Congress Cataloging-in-Publication Data

Breast cancer : a psychological treatment manual / Sandra Haber
   editor.
     p. cm.
   Includes bibliographical references and index
   ISBN 0-8261-8790-0
   1. Breast—Cancer—Psychological aspects. 2. Psychotherapy.
   I. Haber, Sandra
RC280.B8B6656 1994
616.99'449'0019—dc20
                                                94-35284
                                                CIP

Printed in the United States of America

Contents

vi • Contents

Section V   Interventions and Resources

Contributor Biographies

Sandra Haber, PhD, is a psychologist in private practice in New York City and an Associate Clinical Professor of psychology at the Derner Institute of Adelphi University where she teaches and supervises doctoral students in psychooncology. Dr. Haber provides continuing education workshops for psychologists on the psychological treatment of cancer and designs psychological intervention programs for the American Cancer Society and Winthrop University Hospital. In addition to *Breast Cancer: A Psychological Treatment Manual*, Dr. Haber is the co-author of *When Someone You Love Has Prostate Cancer: A Guide For Women and The Men They Love*. Dr. Haber was elected Distinguished Psychologist of the Year for 1993 by the Division of Independent Practice of the American Psychological Association for her contributions in the field of psychooncology.

Catherine Acuff, PhD, is an Associate Professor of clinical psychology at the Graduate Institute of Professional Psychology, University of Hartford. She is past President of the Connecticut Psychological Association and a past Chair of the National Association of Lesbian and Gay Psychologists. She is a proud recipient of the Connecticut Psychological Association's Award for Outstanding Professional Contributions to Psychology in the Public Interest. In addition to teaching and professional activities she has an independent practice in Windsor, Connecticut.

Lauren Ayers, PhD, is a psychologist in private practice in Albany, New York, and is the author of *Teenage Girls: A Parent's Survival Manual*, and *The Answer is Within You: Psychology, Women's Friendships & Breast Cancer*.

Esther Lerman Freeman, PsyD, maintains a private practice in Virginia Beach, Virginia. As a member of the Virginia Beach General Hospital Sleep Disorder Team, Trauma Service, and Medical Advisory Board of the Diabetes Treatment Center, she has a specialty in treating medically ill and traumatically injured patients, health care providers, and their families.

Carol Goodheart, EdD, is a psychologist and psychoanalyst in private practice in New Jersey, a Clinical Supervisor for the Graduate School of Applied and Professional Psychology at Rutgers University, and on the faculty of the Institute for Psychoanalysis and Psychotherapy of New Jersey. Long interested in the association between physical and psychological processes, Dr. Goodheart teaches, writes, and does psychotherapy with people who have medical problems. Her current writing project is on the Psychological Treatment of Patients with Chronic Fluctuating Physical Illnesses.

Christine C. Kieffer, PhD, is a clinical psychologist on the adjunct staff at Children's Memorial Hospital and is also on the clinical faculty at Northwestern University Medical School. Dr. Kieffer is a past President of the Illinois Group Psychotherapy Society and formerly directed the IGPS Post-Graduate Training Program. She serves on the Foundation Board of the American Group Psychotherapy Association and has written numerous papers on women's issues and group psychotherapy. Dr. Kieffer maintains a private practice in Chicago.

Louise B. Lubin, PhD, is a licensed clinical psychologist in private practice in Norfolk, Virginia. She works with individuals with life-threatening illnesses and their families, exploring the relationship of the mind and body and physical disease. She continues to work with and learn from women with breast cancer as an individual, group therapist, and community speaker.

Susan G. Mikesell, PhD, is a psychologist in private practice in the Washington, D.C. area. With her previous education and training in nursing, she has worked in the area of women's health since she entered private practice in 1982. Her focus includes reproductive health issues with an emphasis on infertility and pregnancy loss. In recent years her interests have included trauma and loss focusing on work with chronic illness, cancer, and abuse. She is certified in clinical hypnosis from the American Society of Clinical Hypnosis.

Michele Siegel, PhD, a graduate of Long Island University and a participant in New York University's Post-Doctoral Program, was a co-founder of Bulimia Treatment Associates in New York City. She was the lead author of *Surviving an Eating Disorder: Strategies for Family and Friends.*

Barbara Rubin Wainrib, EdD, is a clinical psychologist and psychotherapist in private practice in Montreal, Quebec, Canada. She is also an Adjunct Professor in the Department of Counseling Education at McGill University where she teaches crisis intervention processes and psychooncology to graduate students. She has held staff appointments at many McGill University teaching hospitals, including the Allen Memorial Institute and Montreal General Hospital. She is the author of *Gender Issues Across the Life Cycle* and co-author of *When Someone You Love Has Prostate Cancer: A Guide For Women and The Men They Love* and *Crisis Intervention and Trauma Response: Theory and Practice.*

Foreword

This book presents a unique approach to breast cancer. Its editor, Dr. Haber, and her contributors provide guidance for mental health professionals in dealing with clients and friends with breast cancer. We encounter this disease frequently in our offices and in our personal life; we need help in providing advice that assures a safe journey to health or, if not, to "being there" for as long and as sensitively as possible.

As a major contributor to the manual, Michele Siegel, Ph.D., draws on her professional knowledge of and her personal experience with breast cancer. It is from individuals such as Dr. Siegel that we learn how to help others. Her insights and strength are models of successful coping. The dedication of the first edition to her was an appropriate tribute to a thoughtful clinician and a remarkably mature mother and wife, who courageously faced the problems of unrelenting breast cancer.

I am honored to be part of this book, which will bring information and insight to those who deal with the psychological side of breast cancer.

JIMMIE HOLLAND, M.D.
Chief, Psychiatry Service
Wayne E. Chapman Chair of Psychiatric Oncology
Memorial Sloan-Kettering Cancer Center
New York, N.Y.

Preface

Women's career styles are quite different from those of their male colleagues, both in their relationships to each other and in their interrelationships with their families. This manual is more than an edited volume. It is a collaborative venture of ten women psychologists, drawn together by the importance of the topic. It was an extraordinary process, and one that I am grateful for participating in. And in the inevitable interconnection of family and career, I want to acknowledge the significant others in the authors' lives for their tangible and intangible contributions.

SANDRA HABER, PH.D., EDITOR

Acknowledgments

We appreciate the contributions of the following individuals who helped in the production of BREAST CANCER: A PSYCHOLOGICAL TREATMENT MANUAL. Without their time, energy, and support, this manual would not be possible.

Jeannie Beeaff
Sally Berg
Lynn Bonde
Deborah Bowen, PhD
John Paul Crown, MD
Ronald Dannenberg
Ruth Jean Eisenbud, PhD
Albert Ellman, MD
Joyce Ford
Marion Rudin Frank, PhD
Shirley Glass, PhD
William Golden, PhD
Jonathan S. Jacobs, DMD, MD, FACS
Paul Jacobsen, PhD
Susan Jacobstein, LCSW

Rosalind Kleban, CSW
Carolyn Messner, ACSW
Lucille Perrotta, MD
Judy Pollatsek, MA, LICSW
Ethel Pollock, MSLS
Robert Resnick, PhD
Zeev Rosberger, PhD
Renee Royak-Schaler, PhD
Rochelle Sax, ACSW
Louise Silverstein, PhD
T. Richard Saunders, PhD
Irma L. Stahl, ACSW
Margaret Stohner, LCSW
Voorheesville Public Library Staff
Patricia Weeks, RN

Special appreciation is due to **Richard Mikesell, PhD.**
As the 1992 president of the Division of Independent Practice (42) of the American Psychological Association, he provided the enthusiasm and the resources for the development and distribution of this manual.

Dedicated to Michele Siegel

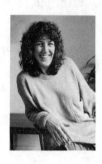

She was a friend, a colleague, and a woman with breast cancer. Her personal and professional insights were invaluable in initiating the writing of this manual. Dr. Siegel died on January 2, 1993. This manual was her last professional involvement and is dedicated to her.

Introduction

A PERSONAL JOURNEY

Seven years ago, my life as a psychologist changed. I had been working with Ann, a 32-year-old patient, for 2 years. Ann came to me with many concerns, one of which was her fear of breast cancer, an illness that she successfully battled prior to her beginning treatment with me. Although she had many family and relationship issues to discuss, her terror of cancer clouded many of our sessions. Visits to her oncologist were the standard procedure for everyday aches and pains. Headaches were brain tumors; backaches were cancer of the spine.

One day, her worst fear came true. She again had cancer.

She died about a year later, possibly of metastasized breast cancer, possibly of a new, unrelated cancer. To this day, I am not sure.

Soon after Ann's death, breast cancer struck again—this time in my best friend. But now, I was a stronger ally. I mastered the medical information, visited the surgeon, discussed treatment options, and waited the endless wait in her hospital room during surgery. I saw the scars following early reconstruction and heard her cry with joy when she heard that her lymph nodes were negative. She recovered, and life is back to normal (or as normal as it can be after you have breast cancer). She learned she could survive. I learned that there is a great deal a psychologist can do in this crisis.

When another longtime friend and colleague, Dr. Michele Siegel, called with a diagnosis of breast cancer, I knew that I could be there for her. Unfortunately, her condition was quite serious. Treatments were more aggressive, and the family situation, with one young child and a newborn, was more complex.

Simultaneously, in a professional capacity, I had been learning more about breast cancer and about the women who were fighting the illness. I was appalled at how much psychological treatment was needed by patients and their families and how few psychologists were actually involved in the treatment of this illness. And so, the idea for a breast cancer manual

TABLE 1 Lifetime Risk Ractor for Developing Breast Cancer at Different Ages (American Cancer Society, 1994)

By age 25:	1 in 19,608
By age 30:	1 in 2,525
By age 35:	1 in 622
By age 40:	1 in 217
By age 45:	1 in 93
By age 50:	1 in 50
By age 55:	1 in 33
By age 60:	1 in 24
By age 65:	1 in 17
By age 70:	1 in 14
By age 75:	1 in 11
By age 80:	1 in 10
By age 85:	1 in 9
By age 90:	1 in 8

was born. *Breast Cancer: A Psychological Treatment Manual* was supported and originally published by The Division of Independent Practice of the American Psychological Association as a way of educating and involving psychologists in the treatment of this illness. Combining friendship and professional interests, Dr. Siegel was invited to be one of the contributors, offering us her experience and insights as a woman, wife, mother, and psychologist with breast cancer.

A STATISTICAL PORTRAIT OF BREAST CANCER

The psychological treatment of breast cancer patients soon became a consuming interest in my life. Breast cancer is an increasingly common illness with 182,000 new diagnoses in 1993 (American Cancer Society, 1993). As noted in Table 1, breast cancer is correlated with age, so that the older woman has an increasingly greater risk of being affected. The common statistic "1 in 9" refers, in fact, to the probability of breast cancer over the course of a woman's lifetime of 85 years. With a life expectancy of 90 years, that probability jumps to 1 in 8.

On the other hand, with the advent of early detection through mammography screening, breast cancer has become a disease that increasingly affects younger women. Breast cancer will strike a sizable percentage of women during the childrearing years and will have an impact on the woman, her partner, and her children.

Breast cancer is a large and growing public health problem in the United States. During the decade of the 1990s, it is estimated that nearly 2 million women will have been diagnosed with the disease and that 460,000 women will have died of it. Between 1950 and 1989, the incidence of breast cancer increased by 53 per cent. The magnitude of this problem and its constant increase over time understandably result in considerable anxiety among all women. (National Cancer Institute, 1993, p. 1)

RISK FACTORS

Although breast cancer has no single known cause, certain risk factors have been identified. Most significant are the age of the woman (see Table 1) and a familial history of breast cancer. The latter factor accounts for 5% of all breast cancers. One in 200 women inherit this genetic factor and face an 80-90% risk of developing breast cancer ("Breast Cancer Research," 1993). At present, research scientists are on the verge of identifying the specific gene for breast cancer, following which genetic counseling for the affected segment of the population is likely to become available.

Surprisingly, high-risk factors such as family history, together with lesser risk factors such as early menarche, late age at menopause, not bearing children or bearing them later in life, account for only a small percentage of the cases of breast cancer; most incidents of breast cancer are not linked to these risk factors.

THE DEVELOPMENT OF PSYCHOONCOLOGY

The psychotherapist can be helpful to patients and family members as they sort through the various treatment decisions for breast cancer. These can include lumpectomy or mastectomy, elective chemotherapy, possible prophylactic mastectomy of the healthy breast, and the option of reconstructive surgery. In addition to the actual treatment choices and an overwhelming anxiety about the cancer, the patient is also faced with a myriad of specialists, which can include an internist or gynecologist, a radiologist, a breast surgeon, an oncologist, a radiation oncologist, and a plastic surgeon. This primarily male medical establishment can intimidate the patient, hamper communication, and feed her sense of passivity and self-doubt, making it difficult to have a voice in decision-making processes.

It is clear that psychological factors affect the appropriateness of patients' decisions and, frequently, their success with treatment. The consideration of these factors has led to the development of a new field of study called psychooncology.

The treatment of cancer has come to be an extremely technical undertaking, based almost entirely within the busiest and most active wards of the hospital, and involving the strenuous efforts of highly specialized professions, each taking his or her responsibility for a share of the patient's problem, but sometimes working at a rather impersonal distance from the patient as an individual. To many patients, stunned by the diagnosis, suffering numerous losses and discomforts, moved from place to place for one procedure after another, the experience is bewildering and frightening. . . . It is only in recent years that oncologists in general have begun to confront squarely the emotional impact of these ordeals and the fact that emotional states play a large role in the tolerability of treatment and, perhaps, in the outcome as well. (Holland and Holland, 1990, v).

This new specialty of oncology, psychooncology, addresses the emotional responses of patients, families, and caretakers (psychosocial) as well as the psychological, social, and behavioral factors that may influence cancer morbidity and mortality.

Breast cancer patients need psychooncological services during diagnosis, treatment, and recovery. Following the initial diagnosis, patients are presented with a series of complicated medical options, all of which are fraught with serious side effects and discomforts. They are asked to come to a decision about their medical care at a time when they are most anxious.

During the treatment and recovery phases, patients and families need allies who can offer support, initiate psychological interventions, and facilitate assertiveness training. The psychotherapist may be called upon to treat the side effects of surgery (scars and loss of the breast) and adjuvant treatments (including feelings about hair loss, fatigue, nausea, and vomiting). General anxiety throughout the course of the illness and fears of recurrence are also common presenting symptoms.

Psychological interventions are not simply ways of helping patients "feel better." Our research colleagues have found that anxiety and treatment side effects have a negative impact on the efficacy of medical interventions and can also result in noncompliance and early withdrawal from treatment (Redd, Andresen, & Minagawa, 1982). Through cognitive-behavioral interventions and supportive techniques, psychologists have been instrumental in helping patients deal with the dysfunctional side effects of medical procedures such as disrupted body image, sexual impairment, anticipatory and posttreatment nausea and vomiting, pain management, and general, overall family crisis (see Golden, Gersh, & Robbins, 1992). Psychological interventions empower patients with an element of self-control in an otherwise out-of-control situation. Psychological interventions promote longer life. Research has found that metastatic breast cancer patients who participated in a support group lived 18 months longer than those who did not (Spiegel, Bloom, Kraemer, & Gottheil, 1989). Research on psychoneuroimmunology has found that psychological interventions affect the immune system in a measurable, though still uncertain, manner. (Anderson, Kiecolt-Glaser, & Glaser, et al., 1994; Fawzi, et al., 1990; Kiecolt-Glaser, et al., 1987).

The psychotherapist can also be helpful in working with the frequently neglected secondary patients—the partner, children, and parents of the breast cancer patient. Although breast cancer has become a publicly acknowledged illness during the past decade, we still find that the families of breast cancer patients suffer in relative obscurity and neglect. The psychological treatment for breast cancer should routinely include interventions for both the patient and family. Partners and children will often require support for legitimizing their needs.

Financial stress, transportation needs, and child care arrangements are some of the issues facing the families of breast cancer patients. Frequently, the ambience in the home changes as the healthy spouse assumes a double workload, and the focus of attention is shifted from the children to the sick parent. The overall neglect of psychological issues in children of breast cancer patients can place these children at psychological risk.

CLINICAL EXAMPLES

Patient 1

Karen, a 46-year-old physician and single mother, was diagnosed with early-stage breast cancer. She had been given a choice between a lumpectomy with radiation or a simple mastectomy. In her case, as in many cases, these treatments yield medically equivalent outcomes. The decision, therefore, was a personal one. At first, the lumpectomy, typically causing only minimal changes to the breast, had enormous appeal. She was, however, deterred by the anticipation of fatiguing and time-consuming daily radiation treatments. Further exploration revealed that she had concerns about possible long-term effects of radiation and continued anxiety about a recurrence. Karen felt that if she had a recurrence, it might manifest itself as a late-stage, advanced tumor. She was afraid of jeopardizing her life and her son's well-being. She began to consider a double mastectomy as both a treatment and prophylactic measure.

Throughout the decision-making process, she faced concerns about physical disfigurement and loss of her sense of femininity. The possibility of immediate reconstruction helped her to feel better about her choice. After some discussion, she concluded that peace of mind by "having it all out" had greater appeal. She opted for a bilateral mastectomy with immediate reconstruction and remains comfortable with her decision at this time, 4 years later.

Patient 2

Sara was a 39-year-old woman who was diagnosed with early-stage breast cancer. Complicating the diagnosis was the fact that Sara was 8 months pregnant with her second child. Having lost her mother to cancer when she was 13, Sara was terrified of leaving her children motherless. We needed to control her anxiety so that Sara could gather information and make a rational decision about treatment. Although she was able to make a choice about mastectomy and reconstruction, she was unprepared for her disappointment in the reconstructed breast. This breast was somewhat smaller and considerably more uplifted than her natural breast. The mismatched breasts raised issues of body image, self-esteem, and femininity for Sara. Although cosmetic surgery was a medical option, Sara chose, through psychotherapy, to come to terms with the physical limitations.

Issues involving her husband's anxiety and the needs of her child and infant were also a part of treatment.

Patient 3

Frank was a 48-year-old man whose wife was dying of metastatic breast cancer. Facing the dual role of father and mother to his two preschool children, Frank was alternately saddened and angered by the circumstances of his life.

Frank required support and the opportunity to focus on his feelings. He also needed education and answers. Issues of psychological significance such as childcare arrangements, sleep disturbances, and communicating with preschool teachers, as well as the daily concerns of food preparation, shopping for clothes, and bathtime rituals were discussed.

The psychotherapy session was the only place where Frank's concerns could be addressed. Daily life was consumed with the needs of his dying wife, children, and business.

Patient 4

Sue was a single 37-year-old woman who was referred for psychotherapy following her breast surgery and during her radiation treatments. She was experiencing queasiness, fatigue, and anxiety. It took her 3 days to recover from her radiation treatments, and she experienced a "not me" feeling the entire time.

As part of an empowerment exercise, Sue focused on her identity before the onset of breast cancer. She was an athletic woman in vigorous health. She liked riding horses and long distance running. These positive experiences of Sue's past successes were used in therapy. For example, in learning to ride a horse she had experienced feelings of soreness, discomfort, and fatigue, as well as wonderful exhilaration. She also remembered that when running long-distance marathons, she felt queasy, dehydrated, and exhausted, as well as victorious.

Using hypnosis, we set about our work "reframing" Sue's radiation treatments. The feelings she experienced were familiar to her, so rather than associating them with the negatives of "cancer patient," work was done on strengthening these same associations to her previous feelings of success and winning. Reminding her of the familiarity of these feelings and the fact that she was winning the battle with her cancer helped reduce her anxiety during subsequent treatments.

TOWARDS THE FUTURE

These are but a few examples of breast cancer patients and their partners who seek psychological treatment. Throughout the pages of this manual, you will hear their voices as well as those of the therapists who treat them.

Unfortunately, despite modern disclaimers, mind-body dualism in the treatment of breast cancer is very much alive. Psychological interventions are usually an afterthought, offered well after the treatment regimen has been completed, and then only if the patient is actively symptomatic. As long as such dualism prevails, psychological services will not have their rightful place as a part of the usual and customary standard of care. As you journey through this Manual, I hope you will join us in offering psychological services to the patients and families who so valiantly battle with this illness.

REFERENCES

American Cancer Society. (1993). *Cancer facts and figures—1993*.

American Cancer Society. (1994). *Cancer statistics—1994*.

Anderson, B.C., Kiecolt-Glaser, J.K., & Glaser, R. (1994). A biobehavioral model of cancer stress and disease course. *American Psychologist, 49(5)*, 389-404.

Breast cancer research: A special report. (1993). *Science, 259*, 618-629.

Fawzi, F., Kemeny, M., Fawzy, N., Elashoff, R., Mortron, D., Cousins, N., & Fahey, J. (1990). A structured psychiatric intervention for cancer patients, II: Changes over time in immunological measures. *Archives of General Psychiatry, 47*, 729–795.

Golden, W.L., Gersh, W., & Bobbins, D.M. (1992). *Psychological treatment of cancer patients: A cognitive behavioral approach*. Boston: Allyn and Bacon.

Haber, S. (Ed.). (1993). *Breast Cancer: A Psychological Treatment Manual*. Scottsdale: Division of Independent Practice, American Psychological Association.

Holland, J.C., & Rowland, J.H. (1990). *Handbook of Psychooncology*. New York: Oxford University Press, Preface, v.

Kiecolt-Glazer, J., Glaser, R., Dyer, C., Shuttleworth, E., Ogrocki, P., & Speicher, C. (1987). Chronic stress and immunity in family caregivers of Alzheimer's disease victims. *Psychosomatic Medicine, 49,* 523–535.

National Institutes of Health. *Breast Cancer: A National Strategy. A Report to the Nation*, October, 1993.

Redd, W.H., Andresen, G.V., & Minagawa, R.Y. (1982). Hypnotic control of anticipatory emesis in patients receiving cancer chemotherapy. *Journal of Counseling and Clinical Psychology, 50* (1), 14-19.

Spiegel, D., Bloom, J., Kraemer, H., & Gottheil, E. (1989). Effect of psychosocial treatment on survival of patients with metastasis breast cancer. *The Lancet, 8668,* 888-891.

Section I.

Medical Aspects of Breast Cancer

Chapter 1

MEDICAL TREATMENT OF BREAST CANCER

"What is there possibly left for us to be afraid of, after we have dealt face to face with death and not embraced it? Once I accept the existence of dying, as a life process, who can ever have power over me again?"

(Audrey Lourde, 1980, p. 25)

A diagnosis of breast cancer frequently elicits reactions of shock and disbelief, as well as feelings of fear and anxiety. During this initial period of shock, the woman is asked to assimilate, simultaneously, a great deal of medical information, so that she can select an appropriate course of treatment. The patient often has a number of choices to make. Understanding the specific procedures as well as sorting through her feelings are of critical importance.

By having a working knowledge of the medical issues the patient will face, the psychologist can support the patient emotionally, facilitate decision making during the course of treatment, and function as a liasion between the patient and her physician. Familiarity with medical issues makes it easier for the psychologist to dispel fears, anxieties, and myths and to stay focused on the individual's psychological reaction without becoming distracted or overwhelmed by the medical component. Medical terms appearing in this section are defined in the glossary (Chapter 15).

☞ *"During the diagnostic workup period, the woman must cope simultaneously with the need to keep her distressing emotions of anxiety and fear within tolerable limits while making the difficult decisions about treatment for a disease that she knows may be fatal. To accomplish this, she must assimilate new medical information that, in itself, produces anxiety."*

(Rolland & Holland, 1990, p. 190)

Diagnosis

■ *MAMMOGRAM* – A mammogram is an x-ray of the soft tissue in the breast. A mammogram may be ordered when a woman or her physician has discovered a sign or symptom that alerts either of them to the possibility of breast cancer, or, it may be done as a routine screening. Mammograms can detect small lesions before they can be detected by touch. However, the results of a mammogram are not foolproof. Both false positives and false negatives can occur, and about "ten to fifteen percent of the time, a malignant lump will not show up on a mammogram. (Hirshaut & Pressman, 1992, p. 64.)" Clearly, not all cancers can be detected early.

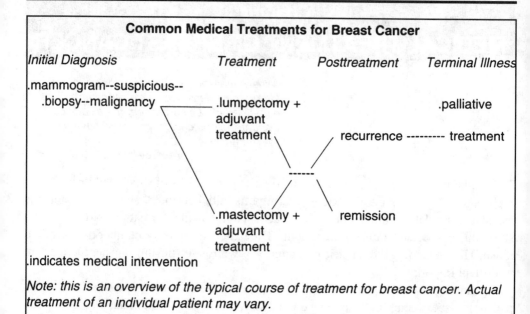

Common Medical Treatments for Breast Cancer

Initial Diagnosis	Treatment	Posttreatment	Terminal Illness

.mammogram--suspicious--
.biopsy--malignancy

.lumpectomy +
adjuvant
treatment

recurrence --------- treatment

.palliative

.mastectomy +
adjuvant
treatment

remission

.indicates medical intervention

Note: this is an overview of the typical course of treatment for breast cancer. Actual treatment of an individual patient may vary.

☞ Although the mammogram is the most sensitive device we have for detecting early breast cancer, a startling 75% of malignant lumps are found by women themselves (Hirshaut & Pressman, 1992). Statistics such as these have led the National Cancer Institute to recommend a three-part program for preventing breast cancer. This program, detailed in a free brochure, consists of breast self examination, breast examination by a health professional, and regular mammograms. Beginning at age 40, all women should have a mammogram every one or two years. When a woman reaches age 50, the frequency should be once a year. (National Cancer Institute, 1990a)

■ **BIOPSY –** The woman is referred to a surgeon or breast specialist who will often perform some type of a biopsy. Biopsies can be performed as either a one-step or two-step procedure. In the one-step procedure, the woman is treated immediately if the biopsy indicates cancer (e.g. with lumpectomy or mastectomy). In the more common two step procedure, the biopsy comprises the first step, and, if cancer is found, subsequent surgery is done in a second, separate operation.

Biopsies range from fine-needle aspiration to excisional biopsy. As in all of the subsequent medical interventions reviewed, there are a number of different possible procedures for the same problem. Each has its strengths and limitations as well as its range of effectiveness.

• *Fine needle aspiration* — A fine needle aspiration is one kind of biopsy often used to differentiate a cystic mass from a tumor. This procedure answers the question of malignancy relatively quickly and does not require surgery. The problem is that it is most accurate when positive. In other words, if the findings are negative, the patient may still have cancer.

• ***Tru-cut needle biopsy*** — The second type of biopsy is a tru-cut needle biopsy which removes a core of cells. It, too, is a non-surgical procedure and it is accurate. The problem is that it is only feasible on certain kinds of lumps and does not give hormone receptor information (though this can be supplied by another test.) The hormone receptor information is important for treatment and will be discussed later.

• ***Incisional biopsy*** — An incisional biopsy removes a wedge of tissue under local anesthetic. Its use is only appropriate with certain types of tumors, and it may be used if the breast lump is large.

• ***Excisional biopsy*** — The area of concern or the whole lump is removed. This is what most surgeons mean by a biopsy. Depending on the size of the lump, this may or may not result in changes in the shape of the breast. The appearance of the breast following surgery should be discussed by the patient ahead of time with the surgeon.

■ *PATHOLOGY* – The pathologist analyzes the biopsy tissue and notes whether or not breast cancer is present and, if it is present, what kind of cancer it is. The frozen section procedure takes just a few minutes and involves looking at thin slices of frozen tissue under a microscope to determine if cancer is present. A permanent section procedure is a more detailed study and takes a few days to assess.

• ***Invasive vs. non-invasive*** — A determination is made as to whether or not the cancer is invasive (spreading) or non-invasive. The non-invasive cancers are sometimes referred to as pre-cancers (ie. ductal carcinoma or carcinoma *in situ*).

• **Staging of the tumor** — The cancer is evaluated or staged by three criteria referred to as the TNM system (tumor, nodes, metastasis). These criteria are: the size of the tumor, the spread of the cancer to the lymph nodes, and the presence of metastasis. Stages are numbered from 0-4, with the higher number being more serious. Cancer cells that are Stage 0, 1, or 2 are most responsive to treatment.

During the staging process, there is also an attempt to ascertain whether the cancer cells are likely to divide aggressively and therefore to spread more quickly. The presence of cancer cells in the blood or lymphatic vessels determines the likelihood of metastasis. However, lymph node evaluation is not foolproof. In cases of invasive carcinoma, 20-30% of breast cancers will spread even though the nodes are negative. The pathologist also determines if there is cancer at the edges of the tissues that were removed (again indicating likelihood of spread).

☞ Patients react to the staging of the tumor in a variety of ways. Some women show limited interest in their diagnosis. Other patients thoroughly investigate their diagnosis. For patients with advanced tumors, the discovery of information on survival rates may be particularly frightening. The stage of the cancer and the survival rate are useful in determining an appropriate course of treatment. These data can also be used to balance treatment options against quality-of-life issues.

The psychologist can help these patients understand that survival rates are based on large numbers of women; the individual woman may or may not fall within the actual survival statistic. **The survival rates are presented here solely to further the psychologist's understanding of the disease and to facilitate the psychologist's work with the medical treatment team. This information is not intended to be given by the psychologist to the patient.**

Stage of Tumor	% of women who survive beyond 5 years
0	> 95
1	85
2	66
3	41
4	10

(National Cancer Institute, 1991)

• **Estrogen receptors** — An estrogen receptor test can also be performed on the biopsy material to determine responsiveness to specific treatments. If the tumor is positive for estrogen receptors, it may well be sensitive to and can be treated with hormones.

Treatment

Treatments can be either local (to the breast itself) or systemic (to the whole body).

■ *LOCAL SURGICAL TREATMENTS* – Surgically, a lumpectomy or mastectomy, each with its relative advantages and disadvantages may be performed. At present, these procedures are considered to have roughly equivalent medical outcomes for many early types of breast cancer.

• *Lumpectomy* — In this procedure, the surgeon removes the breast lump and a sampling of lymph nodes under the arm. The primary advantage of this procedure is that it is usually less disfiguring than a mastectomy. However, there often remains a concern that the breast cancer may reemerge and possibly not be caught as easily. Following a lumpectomy, hormone or chemotherapy may be administered. In addition, radiation, a local adjuvant treatment, is almost always given to increase the effectiveness of surgery (Hirshaut and Pressman, 1992).

In radiation therapy, high-energy x-rays are aimed at the breast, chest wall and sometimes at nearby areas that still contain lymph nodes, to destroy cancer cells. Identifying marks are drawn on the skin to specify the target area. Treatments are usually given 5 days a week, for about 5 weeks. The prolonged treatment period, giving minimal radiation each day, protects the normal body tissue from damage. Radiation treatments are not painful, but can cause intense fatigue and some skin changes as well as the personal complications created by the length, cost, and availability of treatment.

> ☞ *Many women will be asked to choose between a lumpectomy and a mastectomy, because the medical results in some cases will be equivalent. The particular decision reached will be different for each woman. Factors such as availability and time required for radiation treatments enter into the lumpectomy option; possibility of reconstruction and degree to which the breast are an integral part of the woman's sexuality and identity are considerations in the mastectomy procedure.*
>
> *"Sometimes a patient asks me what I'd do if I had breast cancer. I never tell her. I couldn't, because what I think I'd do now might be different from what I'd actually do if I were faced with the reality. But even if I did know, what difference would it make? My choice would be based on who I am—my values, my feelings about my body, my priorities, my neuroses. It would only be valid for me. My patient comes to me for my medical expertise, but **she** is the expert on herself."*
>
> *(Love, 1990, p. 265)*

• *Mastectomy* — A modified radical mastectomy (the most common procedure) involves the removal of the breast and the lymph nodes, but leaves the muscles intact. The mastectomy involves greater alteration to a woman's physical appearance than a lumpectomy, but puts the question of recurrence of breast cancer to rest. You cannot develop breast cancer if you do not have breasts. However, recurrence at the site of the excision, as well as metastasis or spread of breast cancer to other organs, is still possible.

• *Breast reconstruction* — The topic of mastectomy would be incomplete without some mention of breast reconstruction (see photos pp. 8-9). Frequently, the patient may have the option to select surgical reconstruction of her breast. This may be done at the time of the mastectomy and is often a great relief to the patient. Reconstruction may also be done at a later date. The timing of the decision depends on the stage of the cancer, the preference of the patient, and the particular surgeon's recommendations. The reconstruction may involve a silicone or saline implant below the pectoralis muscle, or the use of the abdominal muscle and fat tissue to recreate the breast mound (a TRAM-flap or Transverse Rectus Abdominus Myocutaneous).

At a later time, the nipple may then either be created by using pigmented tissue from other parts of the body or by tattooing a nipple on the breast mound. If there has been a radical mastectomy (more prevalent in the past and included the removal of the

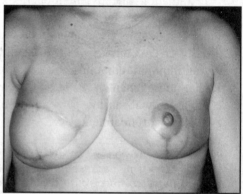

Patient A
TRAM reconstruction of right breast with left breast reduction

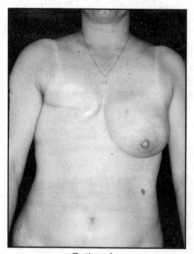

Patient A
Right modified radical mastectomy (with no reconstruction)

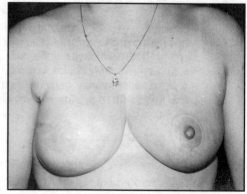

Patient A
Post-nipple reconstruction on right breast

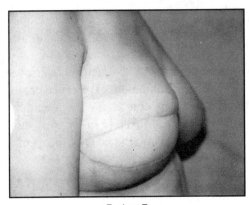

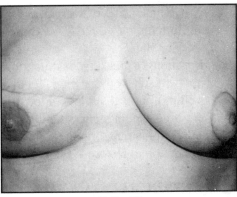

Patient B
Latissimus dorsi *reconstruction of right breast*

Patient B
Nipple reconstruction and left mastopexy (breast lift)

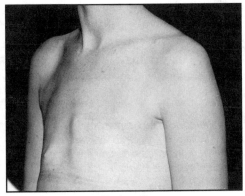

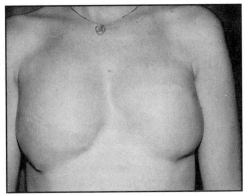

Patient C
Post bilateral simple mastectomies

Patient C
Bilateral tissue expanders fully inflated with saline

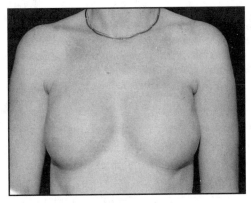

Patient C
Subpectoral bilateral implants (after tissue expansion)

Photos courtesy of Jonathan S. Jacobs, D.M.D., M.D., F.A.C.S.

breast, lymph nodes of the arm, and muscle tissue), a flap may be created on the chest wall from the *latissimus dorsi* muscle in the back. The implant can be positioned under this flap.

Reactions to breast reconstruction are varied. Though some women are overjoyed with the results, others may feel dissatisfied. The woman may experience edema (swelling), as well as loss of local sensation in the reconstructed area. Frequently, there is disappointment when the reconstructed breast is different in size or shape from the remaining breast. In this case, cosmetic surgery on the healthy breast may be an option to restore symmetry to the woman's body.

■ *SYSTEMIC TREATMENTS* – This term refers to treatments to the entire body through the bloodstream. They are classified as either chemotherapy or hormonal therapy.

• *Chemotherapy* — This treatment is offered when the risk of cancer spread is high enough to justify it. Note that age and general health are involved in the determination of feasibility of treatment. Chemotherapy is almost always given to premenopausal women with positive lymph nodes. Chemotherapy may or may not be offered when the lymph nodes are negative. At times, chemotherapy may be combined with hormone therapy.

> ☞ *There are an increasing number of women being offered adjunct chemotherapy with negative nodes. A 1990 National Cancer Institute conference concluded that "although the majority of women with node-negative breast cancer are cured by local treatment, there may be some benefit of systemic therapy in some women with tumors over 1 cm." (Love, 1990, p. 257)*
>
> *"The purpose of chemotherapy or hormone therapy is to prevent the recurrence of cancer. That no one would choose to go through the experience of breast cancer more than once goes without saying. But there is another reality to be faced: it is extremely difficult to cure a recurrence. For that reason, the current consensus is that most patients with breast cancer should receive adjuvant therapy to prevent recurrence...whenever there is an invasive cancer...I do not use chemotherapy or hormone therapy with intraductal or in situ lobular cancer where there is no lymph node involvement, and where the cancer has not spread outside the duct" (Hirshaut & Pressman, 1992, pp.181-182)*

Chemotherapy works by interfering with cell reproduction, so that the cancer cells die. However, chemotherapy is not cell selective, and will destroy all rapidly dividing cells, including hair cells, cells in the intestinal lining, and bone marrow cells. Therefore, chemotherapy is given in cycles in a variety of schedules and drug combinations. The idea is to decrease the total number of cancer cells. Treatments last from 12 weeks to 1 year. Side effects of chemotherapy vary and depend upon the particular drug or combination of drugs, the dosage, route, number of cycles of treatment, and whether they are given with radiotherapy. (Holland & Lesko, 1990). These side effects can include nausea, vomiting, temporary menopause with hot flashes, emotional mood swings, total or partial hair loss (temporary) and vaginal dryness. A discussion of the psychological responses to these side effects can be found in Chapter 3.

• *Autologous Bone Marrow Transplant (ABMT)* — This is a new, presently experimental treatment and is only considered when chemotherapy is clearly insufficient, particularly when cancer cells have extensively metastasized. Standard chemotherapy is limited in strength due to its toxicity to the patient. In other words, standard chemotherapy kills not only cancer cells, but all rapidly growing cells, including bone marrow where white and red blood cells originate. Intense treatment could leave the patient with a weakened immune system, and therefore more susceptible to other diseases.

In ABMT, the bone marrow of the patient is extracted (harvested) for future use if needed. The patient is hospitalized for a period of time. Antibiotics are administered. Megadoses of chemotherapy can be delivered to the patient that are strong enough to wipe out the immune system and the metastasized cancer cells. Until recently, patients were given back their own bone marrow after treatment to facilitate the regrowth of cells. Recent advances have indicated that this step may not be necessary if the patient's own resources can be boosted to facilitate this regrowth process. Side effects of ABMT include increased mortality due to depression of the immune system, large financial expenditure for treatment, and extensive hospitalization time. Note that many insurance companies do not cover experimental treatments.

• *Hormonal therapy* — If the tumor is sensitive to hormones, tamoxifen or hormone therapy can be effective, particularly in the postmenopausal woman. Tamoxifen is an estrogen blocker, and is given in pill form usually twice a day, for 3-5 years. It acts by preventing cell growth. Tamoxifen has fewer side effects when compared to those of standard chemotherapy. At times, it may be given as a combined treatment with chemotherapy.

• *Boosting the immune system* — Crossing the boundary between medical and psychological treatment are complementary treatments that purport to boost the immune system. In the battle of cancer cells *vs.* the immune system, these treatments focus on strengthening the immune system to better fight off the remaining cancer cells. Here lies the interface of medicine and psychology in the subspecialty of psychoneuroimmunology (Bovbjerg, 1990). The central premise of psychoneuroimmunology is that neural activities stimulated by psychosocial factors impact the immune system. There is some clear evidence to support this theory, but the exact processes of influence are, as of now, unknown. A summary of these studies appears in Chapter 13.

Chapter 2

THE RELATIONSHIPS AMONG PATIENT, PHYSICIAN AND PSYCHOLOGIST

"When my doctor stated that I am a demanding patient, I told him that a compliant cancer patient is a dead cancer patient."
(Shirley Glass, 1992, personal communication)

A comprehensive and integrated approach to providing psychological services to the woman with breast cancer requires attention to the system within which she is functioning regarding her medical care. The three primary relationships to consider are the patient-physician, the psychologist-physician, and the patient-psychologist. This last relationship will be explored in Chapter 6.

Of the three relationships, the most significant will usually be the patient-physician relationship (unless the patient's psychotherapy pre-dates the diagnosis of breast cancer). Although the patient-physician relationship does not directly involve the psychologist, the psychologist may help to strengthen and improve this relationship. The psychologist must be mindful of the central role the physician plays in this patient's life at the time of diagnosis and treatment. The patient literally feels that her life is in the doctor's hands. This dependence may be counterproductive, since it will typically cause women to be more affiliative and less assertive at a time when assertive behavior and expression of feelings about cancer may be most helpful (Spiegel, 1990).

The relationship between the psychologist and physician needs to be structured in a collaborative fashion. It is important that clear channels of communication be established, through which necessary information can be shared. This relationship may be very active or may be more distant. What is most important is that the psychologist and the physician have at least one significant interchange of information, during which they can share relevant information and discuss their respective assessments and treatment plans. Once this channel is opened, it may never need to be used again, but it can provide comfort to all concerned (patient, physician, psychologist) that all aspects of care are being attended to, and if any problems arise, there will be easier access. For example, if the patient requires antidepressant medication and the physician is called, the groundwork has been laid and the physician may be more receptive to the psychologist's advice and recommendations.

Conflict and poor communication in any of these three complementary and overlapping relationships can cause anxiety and worry for the patient. Smooth communication and understanding can improve the quality of care and, ultimately, the patient's quality of life after the diagnosis of breast cancer.

Facilitating the Patient-Physician Relationship

■ *INFORMATION* – Help the patient learn how to gather information in an efficient manner during her appointment time with the physician. Suggest that the patient come prepared to appointments with the physician by writing questions down beforehand. If the patient is having difficulty asking or remembering information, it may be helpful to suggest any or all of the following: take notes during the meeting, have a companion accompany the patient to the appointment, bring a tape recorder, or write to the physician ahead of time listing questions.

> ☞ *Here are some basic questions you should expect a physician to answer in a medical situation:*
> * *What is wrong with me?*
> * *What are you prescribing and why?*
> * *Are there alternative methods of treatment?*
> * *What are the benefits of all treatment options?*
> * *What are the risks?*
> * *What should I expect during treatment?*
> * *Are there side effects?*
>
> *(adapted from American Cancer Society, 1987)*

The patient may need additional support and encouragement in knowing how to address difficult and controversial issues with her physician, such as alternative therapies.

■ *TRUST* – It is vital that the patient develop trust with her physician. For the patient, this involves defining her expectations of the physician during treatment. Taking responsibility for her own health, and taking charge of what is under her control, are important in this collaborative relationship. The patient must feel safe communicating her feelings, and she must know that she is heard.

> *Your physician should:*
> * *explain everything*
> * *appreciate what is unique about your illness*
> * *work with your family members*
> * *return your phone calls*
> * *respect appointment times*
> * *choose words carefully*
> * *allow enough time for visits*
> * *be an expert in the field*
> * *consider your needs above everything*
> * *be aware when the relationship is dysfunctional and be willing to improve it, or help you find another physician.*
>
> *(adapted from the National Coalition for Cancer Survivorship)*

■ *SUPPORT* – Discuss the possible benefits/problems in bringing a support person with the patient to the appointment to increase "hearing" information.

■ *ANTICIPATE* – Schedule appointments to allow sufficient time for questions to be answered.

■ *INTERACTION* – Encourage the patient to interact with the physician in an assertive/collaborative fashion. Help the patient practice communicating effectively her anger, fears, and questions.

☞ *"The current climate which dictates that full and complete disclosure of information be given by the doctor, in a uniform manner to all women, fails to take into account the wide variation in women's reactions to the information and the range of ways of dealing with the decisions in treatment..." At least four response types among women (presented to extremes to highlight differences) can be delineated, each of which calls for an intervention or communication approach that is quite different."*

'You decide for me, Doctor.'-typical of the older woman accustomed to accepting authority. She tends to do poorly with physicians that leave decision making entirely in her hands; she experiences this as 'the doctor doesn't know what to do.'

'I demand you do the...procedure'-common among young, well-educated women maintaining an assertive stance. These patients can become adversarial if they feel they are not being heard. They need to be treated as a full participant in all decisions. Detailing all options will be helpful.

'I can't decide'.- Women who are typically overwhelmed by the complexity of the problem and their own anxiety. They do best when slowly walked through each step of the decision-making process.

'Given the opinions, your recommendations and my preferences, I choose...' This is the profile of the mature patient who is able to engage constructively in a thoughtful decision-making process with her physician."

(adapted from Rowland & Holland, 1990, p. 190-192)

■ *RESPONSIBILITY* – Enable the patient to clarify her role in taking responsibility for treatment approaches and choices. Help the patient to see options and choices even if the choices are only slightly different or all the choices are unappealing (e.g., given that she will need chemotherapy, would she prefer to go at the beginning or the end of the week? Does she want blood drawn from her left or right hand?) Encourage some sense of control over the choices that she can make in her treatment.

☞ *"When I went in for my biopsy, the nurse told me to take all of my clothes off. When I asked why I had to take off my underpants, she said, 'Everything needs to be sterile.' I followed orders, and felt terrible because I was exposed in the short gown. During the procedure, it was clear to me that I hadn't needed to take off my underpants. When I went back for the lumpectomy, I bought new underpants, stamped them 'Sterile, do not take off!', and I left them on. The moral of the story is, 'Don't be too compliant.'"*

(Shirley Glass, 1992, personal communication)

■ **SECOND OPINIONS** – The patient may want a second opinion and fear that her physician will feel like she is doubting or rejecting him/her. Aiding the patient in maintaining a good relationship with the physician while she explores all options will be helpful.

Fostering the Physician-Psychologist Relationship

■ **COMMUNICATION WITH THE PHYSICIANS**

• ***Identify the primary provider*** — Clarify who is the primary provider for the patient during the treatment of this illness. There may be a surgeon, oncologist, radiation-oncologist, internist, and others involved in treatment. One of these physicians typically will coordinate the treatment of the specialists. Make sure that is the person you communicate with.

• ***Clarify medical information*** — You need to understand the patient's medical experience— her diagnosis, prognosis, treatment plan, degree of pain associated with the disease, side effects of treatment, probable level of functioning, and the quality of life the patient might be able to expect. Be willing to accept "maybe", "perhaps", and "I don't know", as a response to some questions from the physician. This lack of certainty is part of the disease.

• ***Self-education*** — Know the most common forms of treatment and their side effects. Know the prognosis associated with each stage of the disease. (See chapter 14).

• ***Speak in English*** — (not psychobabble) Be prepared to discuss things that anyone on the health care team can readily understand and will find helpful. Some issues to consider are:
    ... family/social/occupational/situation
    ... previous, if relevant psychological history, e.g., specific anxieties, fears, anger of the patient
    ... beliefs about the illness, whether realistic or unrealistic
    ... psychological strengths and weaknesses in coping with the illness.

• ***Give practical suggestions*** — Some physicians may appreciate practical suggestions that are effective with a particular patient. e.g., "I've noticed Mrs. Smith is calmest when her daughter is present. You might want to consider this if she seems very upset" or, "I find that Mrs. Jones rarely asks for help. When she has called me, it's only been in a dire emergency." Give practical suggestions if possible and appropriate.

■ *AVOIDING CONFLICT WITH THE PHYSICIAN*

• ***Responsibility*** — The physician often feels responsible for the patient's health and may be wary of an unknown professional from a different discipline making unusual or abstract suggestions. Hence, the need to be specific and concrete. The initial contact with the physician may be on the phone or by written communication. If by phone, have an agenda in mind about what you want to relate and what you want to ask. Be sure not to discuss the patient with anyone in the physician's office other than the physician.

• ***Relationship*** — The physician may have a longer established relationship and know more about the patient and the family than you do when you enter the relationship. You need to be sensitive to existing relationships. Respect the relationship between the patient and the physician. Remember that the patient may become increasingly anxious and threatened if there is conflict/tension between the people upon whom she depends for her psychological and physical well-being.

• ***Protocol*** — If the referral was from the physician, make sure to send a written consultation note. If the patient was not physician-referred, you may still want to consider contact (with the patient's consent). You can call before or after sending a report to open communication and establish a working relationship.

This written report should be formal, organized, and helpful. Include a mental status exam, family history, and a statement of the patient's current psychological problems and needs. Clearly state what you will be doing to help the patient within the treatment regimen.

☞ *Consider the following items for inclusion in your letter to the physician:*
- *Thank the physician (if the patient was physician referred). State the date of the initial visit.*
- *Give a brief mental status including how the patient presented herself and the predominant affect demonstrated. Diagnose the patient with particular emphasis on whether psychotropic medication seems appropriate.*
- *Address the patient's perception of the disease and reactions to the diagnosis and treatment.*
- *Give a general plan of psychotherapeutic intervention, with mention of what role, if any, the patient's family will play.*
- *Request ongoing communication as needed to keep a working alliance among all involved parties.*

• *Medication* — Psychotropic medication may be indicated for the patient during the course of her treatment and illness. Determine if the physician typically prescribes anxiolytics and antidepressants or if there is a preference for a psychiatric consultation, should this be necessary.

☞ *Psychologists should be aware that antidepressants can be used effectively to reduce the level of pain in breast cancer patients, even if they are not clinically depressed (Foley, 1985). Also, the tricyclic antidepressants can be particularly useful in the management of sleep disturbances that accompany chronic pain. "The analgesic effects of these medications presumably involve the alteration of the biogenic amines important in pain-modulating systems, particularly serotonin. Those tricyclics with greatest effect on serotonin reuptake, such as amitriptyline and doxepin, are empirically the most useful." (Portenoy & Foley, 1990, p. 378)*

Section II.

Stages of Breast Cancer: Patient's Experience and Treatment

Chapter 3
PSYCHOLOGICAL REACTIONS TO DIAGNOSIS AND TREATMENT

The experience of breast cancer depends not only on the medical prognosis and the extent of treatment, but rests in large part on the woman's prior conceptualizations of the disease and her psychological status. Added to this, and deeply ingrained in our culture, is the concept of individual responsibility for health, with poor health sometimes implying personal causation and weakness. Repressed emotions, depression, poor nutritional intake, and excessive caffeine intake may be seen as explanations for breast cancer. These beliefs are frequent, erroneous, and tend to induce feelings of guilt and blame.

In assessing a patient's psychological status, it is her typical reaction to traumatic events which tends to be the best predictor of how she will experience breast cancer. Since breast cancer occurs in psychologically healthy as well as psychologically ill women, an assessment of the patient's general psychological functioning prior to the illness is always desirable. For most women, regardless of their premorbid level of functioning, the trauma of diagnosis and treatment produces reactions of anxiety, grief, helplessness, and hopelessness (Spiegel, 1990). The psychologist, when possible, should attempt to assess whether the presenting psychological symptoms are a response to the diagnosis of breast cancer, or whether they predate the illness.

☞ *The following is a summary of the psychological reactions to breast cancer and the variables that influence its impact.*

General psychological impact of breast cancer and its treatment are created by:
Psychological discomforts such as depression, anxiety, hostility and fear
Changes in life patterns due to physical discomforts, marital/sexual disruptions, and reduction in activity level
Individual variables that influence intensity and duration of the psychological impact:
Premorbid variables
Patient characteristics: The importance of physical appearance (breast) to patient, age of patient, preoperative expectations
Environmental characteristics: Preoperative preparation by surgeon, quality of marital/sexual relationship
Postmastectomy variables
Patient's particular coping styles: Use, intensity and selectivity of denial and related defenses; search for causes creating self-blame and projection of blame.
Environmental variables
Time elapsed since surgery; availability of support (doctor/surgeon, spouse and family, and other patients); additional medical treatments (radiotherapy and chemotherapy)

(Adapted from Meyerowitz, 1980)

Psychological Reactions to Diagnosis

A diagnosis of breast cancer often comes with no physical symptoms or indicators. A woman may find a lump upon self-examination, or her partner may find one. Discovery of suspicious tissue may also occur during a routine physical exam, or through a mammogram. When breast cancer is diagnosed through a mammogram without a palpable tumor, there is much greater uncertainty for the patient about the accuracy of the diagnosis.

■ *PANIC* – is a common reaction to a breast cancer diagnosis, as a woman may feel trapped in a disease she has long feared. If she has experienced the death of someone close from breast cancer, there may be an immediate identification with this earlier experience, and a revival of emotional responses to the loss of that relationship, as well as heightened fears for her own survival.

Panic reactions which alternate with denial and confusion seem to allow the psyche to gradually absorb the traumatic news, as a woman's mind switches back and forth between rejecting and accepting her new status in bits and pieces. At one moment, she may be terrified and confused, and at another, she may be calm and focused. Over time, an acceptance of the change in health status occurs.

☞ It is helpful to the patient to frame an expectancy of emotional turbulence for the first months, and to discourage her from setting unrealistic goals for her emotional reactions. It also can be helpful to ask her to keep track of how she feels, so that she can begin to predict when she is likely to feel worse. For many women, the period of greatest anxiety and depression is upon waking in the morning, as the news once again becomes real. For other women, the fatigue of evening accentuates these feelings. As a woman ascertains her own emotional pattern, she can normalize the experience, know it will pass, or seek help from significant others at these critical times.

It can also be helpful to ask a patient to list her physical reactions when she is feeling panic, so that she begins to understand the interrelationship of physical symptoms and emotional states. To have an upset stomach, to feel dizzy, or to feel one's heart racing are easier to accept as physical responses to stress, rather than as feared indications of impending loss of control.

Physical exercise, to the level that it is acceptable and safe, can be a useful daily offset to feelings of panic, as patients can release some of the tension that accrues during the crisis, and gain a greater sense of bodily control.

Empathy on the part of the therapist is extremely important, and care should be taken that the patient's feelings are fully heard and accepted with respect. With all of the optimism that could be offered with breast cancer, it is nonetheless a devastating, disfiguring, and at times fatal disease. It may be difficult for the therapist to withhold reassurance and encouragement, but if these are offered too strongly, they may be interpreted as a rejection or trivialization of the patient by the therapist.

■ *GUILT* – seems to be a universal human reaction to trauma and loss. With shock and pain come a drop in the reservoir of good feelings about oneself, so that a woman may find herself asking, "How could this happen to me?" and then, "What caused this to happen?" or "How did I cause this to happen?"

The woman may scrutinize every potentially unhealthy behavior in which she has ever engaged. Significant others in the patient's life may inadvertently contribute to feelings of guilt with questions about smoking, drinking, and dietary behaviors, or breastfeeding decisions. Questioning on the part of others is usually an attempt to decrease their own anxieties, feelings of vulnerability, or impending sense of loss.

> ☞ *"A corollary of the assumption that health is under the individual's control is that the individual is responsible for health. Good health is assumed to result from responsible behavior and bad health from irresponsible behavior. ...The implication of this victim blaming is that the burden of illness is joined by the burden of guilt. If a person can do so much to improve health, bad health can be perceived as a personal or moral failing."*
>
> *(Brownell, 1991, 304-306)*

At other times, manifestations of guilt may not take the expected form. A patient may, for example, be ashamed to tell her mother of her illness, she may have excessive anxiety about her partner's rejecting her for her illness, or she may not want to trouble her doctor with questions because she feels that they are too trivial. The guilty feelings may not be in reference to any particular part of the illness, but may take the form of a general devaluing of one's self, and a difficulty in being appropriately assertive.

> ☞ *If guilt is manifested by low self esteem, it can be helpful to foster experiences which enhance the woman's sense of being valuable, such as visits from beloved friends or caring children.*
>
> *Sometimes women can be more effective in their self-care by first imagining that they are arranging for a daughter's care. Since there is rarely any disapproval attached to a daughter who becomes ill, a patient can be more objective in meeting her own needs, if they are first objectified in this manner.*
>
> *When guilt feelings are specific, for example, that one should have had regular mammograms, it can be helpful to discuss assumptions about one's own behavior. It is a common fantasy that all illness is preventable if one just does the "right" thing. The woman may need to accept herself as both a fallible and mortal human being. Similarly, like humans, mammograms and doctors are fallible. Contrary to popular opinion, detection does not always result in cure. It may be helpful to acknowledge that the patient's behavior was not ideal. And, although she can do little about past behaviors, she can make wiser present and future choices.*
>
> *Often, guilt feelings represent fear of disapproval from important people in the patient's life. Therapists can ask whose face is imagined when the patient feels most guilty, and whose words are heard in one's head criticizing the patient. It is sometimes the case that the patient has felt guilty and uncomfortable most of her adult life, and a diagnosis of breast cancer merely serves to highlight these generalized feelings.*

■ *DIFFICULTY ADAPTING TO ILLNESS* – Typically, diagnosis and treatment begin before a woman feels ill, and consequently she has greater difficulty adapting to what seems to be an invisible illness. Often, in the absence of symptoms, or before beginning treatment, there may be a great deal of confusion since the body has not registered an illness. It is difficult to accept noxious interventions and treatments in the absence of symptoms.

■ *OVERWHELMED* – Newly diagnosed breast cancer patients often feel over-whelmed at the change in their life circumstances, and the myriad of situations that must be addressed. Issues such as choice of medical treatment, problems with husbands and children, debilitating physical changes, fears of mortality, financial burdens, and occupational concerns all bombard the woman within a brief span of time (Loveys & Klaich, 1991).

■ *DISAPPOINTMENT* – Progress in the detection and treatment of breast cancer has been accompanied by the optimistic assumption that the disease is curable if detected early. But mortality from breast cancer remains high, even with significant advances in medical treatment. Breast cancer is probably better conceptualized as a disease that is chronic, rather than acute. Recurrences, albeit treatable, are common.

Psychological Impact of Medical Treatments

Cancer patients' anxiety levels during the course of the disease are typically related to the presence of physical symptoms, rather than to actual risk or physician information. Physical symptoms may be the by-product of cancer, a side effect of treatment, or triggered by psychological reactions. Included in this last category are classically conditioned responses to cues such as the treating physician, the hospital where treatment was given, certain types of food, or the treating psychologist.

> ☞ *Memorial Sloan-Kettering Cancer Center in New York City has recently added a new facility designed to reduce the anxiety inherent in breast cancer diagnosis and treatment. The Center provides breast cancer patients, or those at increased risk for this disease, with diagnostic tests, personal counseling, treatment, rehabilitative servies, and even fitting of prostheses. "While the multidisciplinary approach to breast-cancer treatment is extremely beneficial to the patient, maneuvering within the system has created hardships for many women. The process of going to different locations, undergoing multiple tests and examinations, awaiting diagnosis, and coordinating information from different sources can place excessive physical, mental, and financial demands upon the patient...(Additionally), those who have appointments for counseling about their risk or about prevention can be spared the anxiety they might feel upon visiting a cancer hospital."*
>
> *(Memorial Sloan-Kettering Fact Sheet, 1992, p. 2)*

■ SURGERY

• **Decision-making** — Surgical treatment involves a number of decisions for the patient, including lumpectomy *vs* mastectomy, adjuvant chemotherapy *vs* no chemotherapy, and timing of surgery within the fertility cycle. Unfortunately, choice implies control, so that some women experience more self-blame for unfortunate outcomes.

> ☞ *"In this zeitgeist of patient as consumer the medical patient is asked to make active treatment decisions. While I understand the benefits of this and how in many ways it is preferable to the old 'Doctor is God and Patient is Passive Recipient' it is not without its problems. I found it painfully difficult to discuss and consider medical options without any expertise in the medical field. I was asked to make decisions about things of which I have no knowledge. I was steadfast in my refusal to make decisions out of fear. This meant I needed a tremendous amount of information and I didn't have much time. Whatever I chose, I needed to extricate the tumor quickly. I had...my friend, my internist friend, a very patient surgeon, and many devoted friends and family. What do others do?"*
>
> *(Siegel, 1991, p. 5)*

• **Reactions to mastectomy vs. lumpectomy** — In Rowland and Holland's (1990) summary of the psychological responses to surgery, mastectomy patients appear to experience more depression and greater difficulty with sexuality, body image, and female identity, than do lumpectomy patients. This latter group appeared to retain their feelings of femininity and attractiveness, and were more open in discussing their illness. In both groups, marital adjustment was about equal.

Many patients mistakenly assume that surgical treatment will only affect the body. They are generally reluctant to mention emotional issues and problems to the surgical staff, often assuming that psychological problems are an indication of their own inadequacy in dealing with the disease.

■ CHEMOTHERAPY

• **Medical experience** — The experience of chemotherapy can depend, in part, upon whether chemotherapy is part of the initial treatment plan, or if it is used to treat a recurrence. In the latter case, patients who receive chemotherapy for a second time may have considerably more stress, because a relapse is experienced as more devastating than an initial diagnosis. During chemotherapy, these patients generally interpret physical symptoms as indicative of disease progression, while first-time patients interpret them as side effects of treatment.

Although different treatments may produce various side effects, the usual range can include nausea, vomiting, weight gain, hot flashes, mood swings, and hair loss. In a review on the general side effects of chemotherapy (Holland & Lesko, 1990), the most common side effects noted by patients were hair loss (84%), nausea and vomiting (71%) and tiredness and/or weakness (70%).

- *Emotional experience* — In addition to physical side effects, there are emotional reactions to the experience of chemotherapy. For example, Ganz, Polinsky, Schag, and Heinrich, (1989) compared breast cancer patients with and without adjuvant chemotherapy one month after surgery. They found that chemotherapy treatment increased the levels of anxiety, depression, and fear. Similarly, Meyerowitz, Watkins, and Sparks (1983) in a two year follow-up study on adjuvant chemotherapy, found that 44% of the patients continued to experience long term disruption in their lives.

These studies, however, do not convey the quality of the individual's emotional experience. Michele Siegel (1992, personal communication), in commenting on her experience as a cancer patient, noted that although she was typically prepared for the physical side effects of chemotherapy, she was rarely prepared for the emotional experience. "Unfortunately, in their focus on survival, oncologists can minimize the psychological experience and the side effects of treatment can be underplayed." For example, vomiting is an anticipated physical side effect of chemotherapy, but the actual experience of vomiting can include feelings of shame, embarrassment, dependency, panic, and unattractiveness. The patient is often unprepared for these emotional responses.

Similarly, many women know that chemotherapy can result in hair loss. Yet, despite this knowledge, the actual experience of hair loss can be devastating.

> ☞ *"Losing my hair was the greatest of the many narcissistic injuries. It changes what you look like when you look in the mirror. When a woman looks in the mirror and sees someone she doesn't know—that takes a lot of getting used to. Even if I lived alone, I wouldn't have walked around without a wig...The best thing to do is to get a good wig, before you lose your hair. The quality of the wig is all important. You should feel like you look good in the wig..." (Michele Siegel, 1992, personal communication)*
>
> *Editors note: referrals to wig makers and hairdressers who work with chemotherapy patients can be obtained from oncological nurses and the local American Cancer Society.*

Other emotional reactions are based on specific beliefs about the side effects of chemotherapy. Some women feel that they should be able to control side effects by mental power or a positive attitude. They feel guilty or inadequate when they are unable to do so. Other women worry that the treatment is not working if they do not experience strong side effects. These different levels of understanding and misunderstanding contribute to the emotional reactions during treatment.

■ *RADIATION* – Radiation therapy may have aversive circumstances surrounding its use, as with the very loud noise made by the Betatron, a radiation delivering instrument. Fear and anxiety may be conditioned responses that emerge from this treatment. Other psychological reactions include depression and social withdrawal. Physical side effects of radiation treatment can include debilitating fatigue and skin changes.

Radiation therapy is typically given five days a week for about five weeks. Therefore, the inconvenience and expense of daily commuting to and from treatments often create additional anxieties about transportation, work schedules, and childcare.

■ *AUTOLOGOUS BONE MARROW TRANSPLANT (ABMT)* – Although reports of medical effectiveness for autologous bone marrow transplants are encouraging (Lichtin, Weick, Andresen, Burwell, Sands, Murar, Bauer, Fishleder, Green, and Bolwell, 1991; Gingrich, Burns, Wen, and Clamon, 1991), this form of treatment is still too new to assess its psychological impact. It does appear to create psychological stressors due to the lengthy antiseptic isolation of the patient and the high financial cost of the procedure.

☞ *"When they told me that it was my best shot at a "cure" I was paralyzed with fear. I had never heard of a bone marrow transplant and it seemed ominous indeed...My husband and I were numb with fear. Death rates from the treatment? Now we were in a different ballpark. I had never considered hospitalization as a part of the treatment plan, and now one to two months seemed a given.*

...I had to qualify for a treatment program because they were all part of research studies. I had to have the right amount of the disease for their interests. And what about paying? Blue Cross and Blue Shield was refusing to pay saying these treatments were experimental...Could this really be happening to me? I wasn't even forty years old. No one in my family had breast cancer.

....One of the more repugnant experiences of my life was the day I was being admitted... for the mastectomy. We had to stop at a lawyer's office on the way to the hospital to begin a legal proceeding that we hoped would force (our insurance company) to pay for the bone marrow transplant. In the meantime we had to figure out how we would raise the money. We had no equity in our properties and little savings...

I checked into the hospital for my first bone marrow transplant...This began my 36 day hospital stay. During the first nine days I had chemotherapy every other day. Those were like lost days where I was so sedated I slept most of the day....At a certain point two weeks into the hospital stay my counts dropped low enough to prohibit the children from visiting, to protect me from infection. This began the very toughest time psychologically. I was not allowed out of the room except for walks in the corridor with a surgical mask after visiting hours."

(Siegel, 1991, p. 15)

Chapter 4
PSYCHOLOGICAL REACTIONS TO POSTTREATMENT

Reflecting on the emotional aftermath of survival from breast cancer, Rovner (1987) sums up the focus of the experience: "You always are wondering when it will come back" (p. 12).

The research on this stage of breast cancer is focused on survival, as measured by the length of time between initial diagnosis and recurrence. Studies suggest that the aggressiveness of the original tumor, the number of sites, and the type of treatment employed (surgery, radiation, chemotherapy and/or any combination) outweigh the psychological factors as most relevant in determining survival (Watson, 1988). Even in the new area of psychoneuroimmunology, the extent to which the body's defenses can be mobilized against tumor growth and metastasis is linked to the basic tumor and its treatment. Rather than "cure," it is more helpful to consider psychological interventions as contributing to the quality of the woman's life and offering her some control over the disease. The explicit and implicit contract between the psychologist and the patient should reflect this goal.

Clinical Reactions

Breast cancer patients often talk about a shift in emotions once treatment has been completed. Most women eagerly await the end of their treatments. When treatment ends, however, it is typical for anxiety levels to rise. As long as treatment occurs, the patient may have a sense of "doing something" about the cancer. Once treatment is over, the woman is left on her own to deal with the aftermath of the illness. The dominant issues during this period are those of loss, feelings of anger and depression, fears of recurrence, and redefinition of self.

■ *LOSS* – For the posttreatment woman, the experience of loss can come in many forms:

• *The structure and support* that was part of the regular contact with medical personnel during the treatment stage is no longer part of her regular routine. She may experience a loss of this umbrella of protection.

• *The woman experiences a loss of her sense of normalcy* as she discovers that both physically and psychologically, she is different than she was prior to the breast cancer experience.

• *The woman's trust in her bodily experience may be shattered* and this is particularly true for those women who felt physically well and were responsible in their self-care prior to the diagnosis of breast cancer.

- *Loss of or change to the breast* can alter the woman's body image and identity. The symbolic meaning of the breast will vary from woman to woman.

- *The single woman* will be affected in a relationship with new partners. She will again need to learn how and when to expose herself, both emotionally and physically.

- *The working woman* may experience losses on the job. Her employer's knowledge of the breast cancer experience may affect work assignments. Her co-workers may relate to her differently. She may find that her actual capacity to work is diminished, particularly during the course of medical treatment. In considering a new job, she may find that the new employer views her as a liability. She may also experience difficulty in obtaining health care coverage.

- *The married or coupled woman* may experience loss within the partnership. The relationship may not withstand the changes that have taken place over the course of diagnosis and treatment, or the tensions that are reinstated during the posttreatment phase. In a figurative sense, the relationship that the couple once had will never be again.

- *The sexuality of the woman* will often be altered by the breast cancer experience. The woman may experience a changed sexuality as a reaction to mastectomy. She may also experience premenopausal symptoms as a result of medical treatment. Unfortunately, physiological changes that result in disturbances to sexuality are often overlooked or are attributed solely to psychological reactions, rather than to side effects of medical treatment.

> ☞ *Certain chemotherapy agents can adversely affect sexual functioning and desire and interfere with the production of sex hormones. This interference can cause physical changes that make intercourse painful, limit arousal, and inhibit orgasm. These changes are not reversible without hormone replacement. This side effect to chemotherapy is not typically part of the informed consent that the breast cancer client makes at the time of treatment.*
>
> *(Kaplan, 1992)*

- *Fertility* may be affected, depending upon the medical treatment. Some women may experience a permanent impairment of fertility.

  For the pre-menopausal woman without children, this can be particularly devastating. Additionally, even when fertility remains unimpaired, pregnancy may be medically inadvisable.

- *The experience of motherhood* may be changed for the woman who has had breast cancer. The mother's experience of loss varies with the age(s) of her child or children. With young children, she may anticipate the loss of being with them through their growing years. If the children are grown, she risks the loss of enjoying the fruits of the continuity of that relationship.

■ *ANGER AND DEPRESSION* – It is usually when treatment ends that the woman realizes the permanence of these changes and losses. During the treatment period, the emphasis was on physical survival. Now that she has survived, the woman is often surprised and unprepared for the psychological reactions that can occur next. This experience may result in anger or depression. These emotions can be exacerbated if she initially felt responsible for causing the illness. Following treatment, she may again feel responsible for the losses and changes that occurred not only to herself, but to significant others. These reactions can be a normal process in the breast cancer experience.

■ *REDEFINITION OF SELF* – It is in this posttreatment time period that the woman experiences the residual physical and/or emotional effects of treatment. She learns that cancer is a chronic illness, even when the treatment is declared successful. She discovers that her fantasy that once treatment is over she will feel like her pretreatment self is indeed a myth. This myth is can also be fostered by the significant others in the patient's life, leaving her alone to struggle with her changes and losses.

For most women, the intense experience during posttreatment centers on the worry about recurrence. This tends to keep the woman hypervigilant for at least the first five years following treatment. Most women experience marked fears and panic about noncancerous symptoms such as headaches, fever, and pain (Easterling & Leventhal, 1989). This worry and anxiety has the potential to maintain a low-level depression in the posttreatment woman.

■ *CHARACTERISTICS OF SURVIVORS* – Descriptions of psychological factors such as feelings, thoughts, behaviors, and the social environment of the woman with breast cancer have identified some consistent characteristics related to survival (Levy & Wise, 1988).

• *Personal characteristics* — Women surviving recurrence free from breast cancer five to ten years after diagnosis tend to show more intense (though varied) affect.

> ☞ *Patients who showed a "hostile" or "dysphoric" mood and were "unpleasant" in their physicians' eyes were likely to live significantly longer than women who stoically accepted the illness or primarily displayed feelings of helplessness and hopelessness. (Derogatis, Abeloff, & Melisaratos, 1979; Levy & Wise, 1988) Similarly, patients who exhibit information-seeking behavior as well as a fighting spirit as an initial response to breast cancer showed increased survival times. (Nelson, Freidman, Laer, Lane & Smith, 1989)*

• *Social support* — Research on the effects of social support and the prognosis for women with breast cancer indicates consistently positive correlations. Supportive friends and a strong social support network clearly contribute to length of survival. Conversely, social isolation and lack of social support (in addition to apathy and unhappiness) were predictive of a lowering of the natural-killer cells and a poor prognosis in early stage breast cancer (Reynolds & Kaplan, 1986; Levy, Herberman, Maluish, Schlien, & Lippman, 1985; Levy, Herberman, Lippman, & d'Angelo, 1987).

A common misconception is to define social support by the presence of marriage. Research indicates that support may come from relationships other than marriage. In fact, the effect of being married on survival time yields contradictory findings (Spiegel, 1990; Waxler-Morrison, Hislop, Mears, & Kan,1991). For further discussion, consult the section on Husbands and Significant Others.

Treatment Strategies

The woman with breast cancer in the posttreatment stage may enter the psychologist's office through many doors. Sometimes the psychologist's relationship with the patient predates the diagnosis of breast cancer. At other times, the woman may have come to the psychologist to deal with depression or marital difficulties that have occurred following the experience of breast cancer. She may or may not be aware of a relationship between the cancer experience and the presenting issues. Sometimes the woman who is actively being treated for breast cancer is referred to the psychologist by her physician. Regardless of the reason for entering treatment, there are some specific interventions that should be considered for all women in the posttreatment phase of breast cancer.

■ *EDUCATION AND NORMALIZATION* – Normalizing certain psychological responses for women who are in the posttreatment stage of breast cancer is reassuring. The patient can begin to understand normal grief reactions and anticipate changes that will occur. She can be provided with information on support networks (see Chapter 14) that can help her feel less alone in this experience. These groups are typically focused on empowering the woman in work, at home, and with herself.

■ *SHORT-TERM SUPPORT AND COUNSELING* – The psychologist is there to assist the woman in the development of her survival plan. In addition to working through the many issues previously discussed, some women may need help in processing guilt experienced for living through the disease. This may be especially pronounced if others in her family have died of breast cancer. She may also feel guilty for affecting the lives of significant others due to financial burden, increased dependency, or any of the myriad of changes that occurred.

Support for the patient may include the development of new definitions for the meaning and purpose of life, encompassing a definition of self that includes but is not based on the disease. A plan for indefinite vigilance needs to be incorporated into this definition, without the accompanying obsession that is possible.

The psychologist may suggest readings (see Chapter 14) that describe personal experiences with breast cancer. This enables the woman to identify with other breast cancer survivors. Such books are typically helpful for breast cancer patients, but may be especially valuable if the woman is reluctant to participate in a support group.

■ *PSYCHOTHERAPY* – The psychologist can work more directly on psychodynamic issues and behavior change with the posttreatment cancer patient than with the cancer patient who is in a crisis state, whether from a recent diagnosis, current medical treatment, or the experience of a recurrence. As long as there is no recurrence or metastasis of the disease, psychologists can work in their customary ways with the individual woman or the couple who have experienced breast cancer.

The psychodynamic psychotherapist may focus on the reawakening of historical issues that may have formerly been dormant for the breast cancer patient.

☞ *Typical issues for the patient in psychodynamic psychotherapy are:*
- *The end of medical treatment itself can evoke primitive reactions of fear and abandonment.*
- *The normal depressive responses to the losses involved with breast cancer can evoke old patterns of behavior or feelings that may need psychopharmacological intervention.*
- *Women who do not have a well developed sense of self may find the trauma of the breast cancer, its treatment and subsequent recovery threatening to a shaky internal self definition. Issues of femininity, identity, anger and self confidence may concern the patient.*

Chapter 5

RECURRENCE AND TERMINAL ILLNESS

*"Sometimes fear stalks me like another malig-
nancy, sapping energy and power and attention
from my work. A cold becomes sinister; a
cough, lung cancer; a bruise, leukemia."*
(Lourde, 1980, p. 15)

Recurrence, the redevelopment of breast cancer in the breast tissue, is feared most during the first five year post surgical period. Most women remain more vigilant in that early period and feel relatively safe when no recurrence appears in that time frame. Although the five year interval is often used as a benchmark of "cure", it is unrealistic to believe that one is not vulnerable to breast cancer once this period has ended. Frequently, the issue is not whether the patient will have a recurrence, but when she will have a recurrence.

Fear of recurrence and terminal illness is typically greater when there was a metastasis (the development of breast cancer cells in tissue other than the breast) at the time of the original diagnosis. Metastasis may be present at the time of the original diagnosis (e.g., lymph node involvement) or may develop after treatment has been completed. The woman may become aware of the metastasis later, when a lesion is discovered in a new site, such as the bone, brain, or lung. These cancer cells are breast cancer cells in new locations.

When there is metastasis or recurrence, the number of cancer sites involved is the best predictor for length of survival. Both recurrence and metastasis posttreatment signal to the woman that she is facing a shorter life span than she may have come to believe after the initial treatment was completed.

Immediate Reactions to Recurrence

■ **PERSONAL RESPONSIBILITY** – The experience of recurrence may yield a variety of responses. Most often, during the posttreatment period the woman has been doing the best she can to prevent the recurrence of her breast cancer. She may have developed a new dietary and exercise program. She has worked hard on developing relaxation and imagery techniques to enhance her body's healing process. She has diligently followed the physicians' recommendations regarding medications and monitoring. The more control she thought she had with these behaviors, the more vulnerable she may be for feeling responsible (not having done enough or done it right) when the cancer returns.

For other women, especially those who had localized breast cancer, self-care may have been more limited. The patient may have been less careful in self examination or in follow up visits. Frequently, this behavior was an expression of the wish to deny her illness and return to the precancerous period. The experience of recurrence for these women, may be one fraught with guilt and self- blame.

Sometimes, feelings of failure are handled by altering the experience of cancer. Cognitive dissonance (the shift in a belief system to reconcile information) sometimes occurs in cases of recurrence. Patients come to believe that they really did not make their own treatment decision. They may blame the physician and minimize their own responsibility, or they may deny the severity of the recurrence (Wagner & Taylor, 1986).

■ *LOSS OF HOPE* – The woman may believe that the recurrence indicates an imminent death. She may start to withdraw because she has taken the recurrence to mean survival is now at an end. Symptoms of hopelessness may differ. Some women adopt a "winter coat passion" (Pollatsek, 1992). The woman may speak of buying a new winter coat in the middle of summer. This coat is the one she always wanted, but did not need. She has to have it now, before it's "too late". Another expression of hopelessness is giving away belongings, also a signal that the woman has given up hope and believes that life is over.

■ *DENIAL* – The psychological response to a recurrence can be similar to that of the initial disease. The woman may deny the recurrence and delay having the site checked. She may avoid the surgical appointment to have the new lump biopsied. This is the moment that the woman has been anticipating with each breast examination and mammogram. This type of avoidance is associated with "helplessness" that has been correlated with shorter life span after the rediscovery of breast cancer (Levy, 1985). When denial remains the primary response, including a prolonged delay in verification of the new lesion, the woman has more ammunition for feeling responsible for her illness. This may open the door for more intense depression and hopelessness.

■ *GRIEF* – The rapidity with which recurrence turns into terminal illness depends on the aggressiveness of the disease. The psychological transition from recurrence to terminal illness is highly individual. Initially, the grief may be centered on the disappointment in the efforts she has made to foster health and healing. This grief can be short-lived, if the woman can maintain the perspective that life is not yet over. The normal grief reactions including denial, anger, depression, and bargaining all appear at various times throughout this period.

Role of the Psychologist

■ *UNDERSTANDING ONE'S OWN REACTIONS TO DEATH AND DYING* – In order to work effectively with women who are in or approaching the terminal stages of breast cancer, the psychologist needs to be aware of his or her own feelings about death.

☞ In order to be credible as a support structure for the woman, the psychologist needs to know if s/he can be available to the woman in the more debilitating stages of the disease. It is important not to abandon a patient at the last stages of life. Therefore, the psychologist must be able to tolerate his/her own death anxiety. (Further discussion of this topic can be found in Chapter 9.)

Psychologists need to be clear about their own limits before entering into a contract with a patient who has recurrent cancer that is moving toward terminal illness.

The psychologist needs to know how to follow the woman's lead, not intruding too much and not holding back too much. The client's need determines the amount of involvement the psychologist will assume during the actual dying process.

Consultation or supervision with someone who regularly works in the area of death and dying or participation in a peer supervision group can be helpful to the therapist.

Interventions

■ *WORKING WITH DENIAL* – Denial is a defense which will play a role in many patients' reactions to a potentially life-threatening illness. Generally, in the midst of newly acquired information, the woman needs denial to aid her in assimilating the information at a pace she can handle. It is when denial begins to interfere with appropriate decision making about treatment (e.g. blanket refusal to consider treatment options) that it is necessary for the psychologist to begin to address the defense. Denial should be addressed if the therapist believes that medical decisions are being made or avoided based on fears and depression. When working with denial, the psychologist is simultaneously balancing the invitation to look behind the defense, while respecting the woman's right to maintain the defense.

☞ **Addressing Denial**

The psychologist can begin to address denial with questions like:

"What if the lesion (lump) has stray cells that were not removed with surgery?"

"How would you feel about using (or adding) radiation or chemotherapy to lower the chances of the cancer recurring?"

In the terminal stages of the illness, the "what if" questions may revolve more around planning for final events prior to death and goodbyes to family and friends.

The psychologist should pay close attention to the woman's responses. As the patient is able to let go of her defense, the "what if" questions will lead to increased revelation of feelings. If she is unable to relinquish the denial, her responses will be short and somewhat depersonalized.

Allowing Denial

The following is an example of allowing denial with a patient who has a second episode of breast cancer: You notice that your patient keeps referring to it as "small", "minor", or "a new primary lesion" so that she does not have to confront the more frightening implications of a recurrence or metastasis. She is using denial. In this case, it is not important to challenge her definition of the lesion, since it leaves her with hope, a feeling that will be helpful during the possible recurrence and terminal stages of breast cancer. However, any denial around treatment decisions is important to confront, since it can have life-threatening implications for the patient.

Denial vs. Unpopular Decisions

It is important to try to differentiate when a patient has thought through her options and is choosing to forego a treatment based on rational and responsible decision-making. Keep in mind that there are times when a patient's decisions are rational but unpopular with family members. It is important to know what significant family members are aware of with regard to diagnosis, treatment options, and mortality. Secrets between and among family members are common with cancer, particularly in the terminal phase of the illness.

Living wills and right-to-die issues may be important for the patient's consideration at particular times during the treatment. A durable power of attorney is a legal document that, in some form, is recognized in 48 states. Because of the variance from state to state, a local attorney should be consulted for preparation of the document. A durable power-of-attorney for health care can give the person designated as agent the power to make health care decisions. Note that it takes some time to create and execute this document, so it is better if the patient is aware of this option early in her dealings with breast cancer.

• *The ongoing task of the psychologist is to keep hope alive* and although the functional status of cancer patients does not change with counseling in the late stages of the illness, quality of life can be affected (Linn, Linn, & Harris, 1982). Hope changes from "I will beat this" to "I will survive until..." This sentence will end differently as the client's status changes. Initially, the psychologist works on changing the focus from "I will die from this" to "How will I do what I need to do to survive this next treatment or this next stage of the disease?" In order to help the patient reframe hope, the psychologist should be knowledgeable about the progression of the disease once recurrences or metastases appear.

• *Balancing denial and the awareness of inevitable death is stabilizing for the woman* and allows her to consider treatment that could provide her with a more positive experience of death. The client may be afraid to discuss death due to the unexpressed fear that talking about it will make it happen. This belief may be shared by both the patient and her family.

> ☞ *The psychologist can maintain the hope and still explore reactions and feelings about dying by using "what if" questions. For example: What if you do not get better? What are the things that would concern you the most if you do not get better? What if the only difference between you and the rest of the world is that you may have a better idea of* **when** *you will die (rather than if you will die)?*

• *Assist the woman in maintaining her daily structure* and develop a personal plan for action. This gives her a sense of control that fosters hope. Support a positive outlook and a sense of humor which encourages a feeling of being alive.

• *Even if the patient is seeing the psychologist regularly, it is important to have at least one other individual* in whom the woman confides who will give her honest feedback about her reactions to stressful situations. Encourage the maintenance of relationships that involve cooperation and mutual responsiveness. Weisman and Worden (1975) found that individuals who had these kind of relationships, particularly toward the end of their lives, lived longer.

• *A support group* involving other women who are struggling with the terminal stages of breast cancer provides a balance of hope while facing the reality of loss. Spiegel and Yalom (1978) suggest that a major task of a support group for dying patients is to answer the question "What remains of myself when I give up highly valued functions and attributes?" This is an important question to be able to answer to keep hope realistically based for as long as possible.

☞ *INTERVENTION STRATEGIES*

The psychologist starts by redefining help from cure and fixing, to support and witnessing.

Know that physical presence and practical assistance should be offered without the client having to ask.

Offer information and choices to keep the balance between taking over and giving control. Anticipate and help plan for holidays and anniversaries with the client and the survivors.

Expand the concept of normalcy by respecting the self-protective nature of the shock and denial expressed by the client. Reinforce the reality of loss by sensitively using the words death, dying, and suicide (when appropriate). Validate the client's right to a temporary evasion of reality.

Acknowledge hidden grief by giving permission for the expression of pain, helplessness, frustration, fear and hurt caused by loss. These are likely to be expressed in explosive emotions like anger, hate, blame, terror, resentment, rage, and jealousy.

Control, even in the smallest way, should be identified for the client. Support decisions made by providing accurate information and offering choices and alternatives. Hope refocused legitimately enhances this sense of control.

Listen without judgment, retaliation, or argument to strong emotions. This validates them and encourages their expression. Be available to hear the story of her life and her disease, encouraging ways of remembering including photographs, tapes, diaries, and letters.

(adapted from St. Francis Center, 1991)

Section III.

Psychotherapy with the Breast Cancer Patient

Chapter 6

THE PATIENT-PSYCHOLOGIST RELATIONSHIP

The patient-psychologist relationship during the crisis of breast cancer functions in a broader arena than is typical in traditional psychotherapy. To provide quality care, it is important to see ourselves as part of the larger health care "team," both gathering and providing vital information for and with the patient. With the patient's consent, our usual interest in protecting confidentiality at all costs may be best replaced by an attitude of medical and family collaboration. The appropriateness of this exchange will vary at different stages of the illness, so that during remissions or after a "cure," there will often no longer be a reason to share information. If, however, the patient becomes weak or disabled, we may actually need to "talk for them" and make their wishes known.

> ☞ It is important to note that all information shared is done with the patient's knowledge and written consent.

Management Issues

■ *ESTABLISH THE BOUNDARIES* and parameters of the relationship with the patient at the onset of treatment. Keep in mind that scheduling flexibility may be needed due to hospitalization or debilitating physical symptoms. Discriminate between depression and disease-related disability with regard to the patient's attendance at sessions. Sometimes it is necessary to encourage the patient to keep her appointment even if she is not feeling well.

> ☞ "Several issues complicate psychotherapy with cancer patients, requiring a modified approach from the way in which treatments would commonly be carried out with physically healthy patients. The therapist may initially feel as if he or she is 'breaking the rules' learned in supervision doing psychotherapy with healthy individuals...."
>
> *(Massie, Holland, & Straker, 1990, p. 463)*

■ *EXTEND PARAMETERS* but keep in mind boundaries with regard to where one is willing to see the patient. Be aware of your feelings as well as the patient's feelings about hospital or home visitation. It is important to keep in mind when to visit a patient in the hospital. Is the request made by the patient, the physician, or by the family? This also applies to home visitation and phone consultation.

■ *OBTAIN INFORMED CONSENT* to communicate with the patient's physician. Define the limits of the interaction you will have with the physician and communicate this to the patient. Help the patient see that you are part of the total health care team which will play a role in her treatment.

■ *BE PREPARED* to suggest ways of working with the significant others or children of the patient, because these family members are deeply affected by the experience of breast cancer (see Section IV of this manual). Each individual, couple or family may require consultation or treatment. Deciding when to see members of the same family and when to refer them to other therapists will be an important decision during the course of treatment.

■ *DEFINE WHEN BEING "PURELY SUPPORTIVE"* is the appropriate treatment, e.g., for a terminal patient you have been working with in psychotherapy.

■ *IF THE PATIENT DIES* you will need to make a decision about contacting the family and attending the funeral. You may also discuss this with the patient (if they express a wish to discuss this) during the terminal phase of the illness.

> ☞ *Know the community resources that are available in your community. Use the resource numbers listed in the back of this manual to access information about your community. Being part of a larger treatment continuum is central to good psychological care.*

Ongoing Issues in Treatment

■ *ALTERATIONS TO THE BODY* will involve assessing the patient's body image before and after breast surgery. How does the surgery impact on her, and what adjustments has she had to make in her activities, relationships, sexual functioning, dress, and comfort?

These experiences will vary with the specific surgery (lumpectomy, mastectomy, radical mastectomy, or lymph node removal), the previous body image of the patient, the availability of reconstructive breast surgery, and the response of significant others.

■ *SIDE EFFECTS* are a part of any treatment. What are the ones that are most unpleasant for this particular patient? Hair loss from chemotherapy may be more distressing than pain or vomiting. Weight gain may be a worry of some women. Physical restrictions such as not lifting a child may cause anxiety, as can coping with early menopause or menopause-like symptoms.

■ *COPING WITH PAIN* is of critical importance. Is the pain constant or transient? Is it severe or mildly uncomfortable? Does pain interfere with physical or emotional functioning? Is medication needed to reduce the pain?

■ *THE EMOTIONAL EXPERIENCE* of the patient will vary with the stage of the illness, the treatment experience, and the psychological makeup of the individual. The patient who has just received an initial diagnosis will be focused on treatment options and fears around those decisions. Patients with more advanced or recurring breast cancer may be focused on alternative treatments or issues of mortality. The reality of these fears can be assessed by communicating with the medical team. Attempt to understand what information the patient and family have about the illness. Try to determine if the patient has accepted, rejected, or distorted the information given. Is she seen as cooperative with the medical team? Does the family attempt to shield the patient from information she needs to know?

> ☞ *Cancer Care, Inc. offers some suggestions for helping the patient communicate more effectively about cancer pain. Ask the patient to:*
> - *Keep a record of what makes pain better or worse, and when this happens.*
> - *Describe the pain with specific words such as aching, shooting, numbing, or tingling.*
> - *Rate the pain on a 0 to 10 point scale, where 0 indicates no pain and 10 indicates the worst pain imaginable. For children (or non-verbal patients) a picture rating scale can be used with happy, sad and crying faces.*
> - *Rate the pain relief on the same one to ten point scale, prior to and after using medication.*
>
> *(adapted from Cancer Care's Pain Resource Center)*

■ *TREATMENT CHOICES* – are difficult to make, given such issues as the odds of living *vs.* the quality of life. Patients may want to find out how likely they are to have a successful outcome with a given treatment. What does a "successful outcome" mean to this particular patient in terms of time and disability? What are the costs—physical, emotional, and financial—of not having the treatment? Patients must deal with the uncertainty of the future and struggle with the reality that their physicians do not have all the answers.

Psychotherapy When the Patient is in Crisis

During the initial diagnosis of breast cancer, or during periods of recurrence, the therapist will often find that the patient needs more focused and active therapeutic interventions.

> ☞ *"Using a brief therapy crisis intervention model, focus is kept on the illness and present concerns. The therapist first encourages expression of feelings and fears about the illness and its outcome; fears are often considered by the patient to be too painful and too burdensome to reveal to family and friends, and hence the therapy plays a useful role in exploring and exposing the feelings. Support is offered by the therapist, who usually can help the patient see that most concerns are universal."*
>
> *(Massie, et al, 1990, p. 462)*

Whatever your usual treatment orientation— psychoanalytic, cognitive, existential-humanistic, or behavioral— a more active and focused intervention is often needed for the patient with breast cancer, both for those newly diagnosed and those undergoing a recurrence. Even for long-term psychotherapy patients, the diagnosis of breast cancer suggests that the therapist shift modalities to incorporate a more focused approach until the patient is emotionally stable. The change from a more traditional approach is suggested because the diagnosis and recurrence of breast cancer is a threat to the patient's psychological equilibrium and integrity as well as to her life. A focused approach allows the therapist to respond to these threats most effectively by incorporating techniques (if they wish) derived from a wide variety of therapeutic orientations, including cognitive, humanistic, existential and dynamic, any of which may be helpful in this situation. These techniques (see chapter 12) can empower the patient to deal effectively with her life at a time when she is feeling most powerless. A return to the therapist's own modality may occur once the crisis has been overcome.

> ☞ *"When patients experience a remission and health becomes more normal, the confrontation with cancer and death sometimes is an impetus to explore problems that might otherwise have been tolerated...Psychotherapy, begun during cancer treatment, may be the proper place to consider priorities. The format of this therapy should revert to the more usual contract of regular visits in which the therapist takes a less active stance. It is preferable to move closer to the traditional model during any period of remission or when the patient is well enough to benefit from a more exploratory model of psychotherapy."*
>
> *(Massie et al., 1990, p. 464)*

Approaches to the Crisis

Both crisis intervention and short-term dynamic psychotherapy are examples of approaches that offer active, time-limited, focused treatment suitable for the patient with breast cancer. These orientations can be compatible with each other and may also be combined with crisis-specific exercises, cognitive behavioral strategies, and the readings suggested in Chapter 14.

■ *BASICS OF SHORT-TERM DYNAMIC PSYCHOTHERAPY (STDP)* – The independent practitioner working under the constraints of insurance reimbursement or limited family funds may find short-term dynamic psychotherapy cost-effective. Using a time- limited modality, the patient participates in (most typically) 6-30 sessions of face to face, once a week treatment. Psychoanalytic theory underlies this technique, and interventions such as clarification, confrontation of affect, and interpretation may be used. As in all work with breast cancer patients, the goal is to empower the patient, support her through the trauma, and increase her ability to function. The therapist maintains a flexible stance, and evaluates the appropriateness of any suggestion on a case-by-case basis.

However, if the patient becomes more ill with breast cancer, she will need more help, *regardless* of the availability of funds. Under these circumstances, it must be recognized that the woman has a need for on-going, non-time limited support, although the support does not necessarily have to take the form of psychotherapy. The practitioner's decision about the selection of an STDP modality will also be more complicated if the woman has a history of psychopathology.

■ WORKING WITH THE BREAST CANCER PATIENT USING STDP
(as described by Goodheart, 1989)

• ***Limit the focus*** by doing only the piece of therapeutic work that is essential to the patient at this time. Treatment is focused on issues related to breast cancer so as to improve the patient's ability to function.

• ***Provide a supportive holding environment*** which is a "container" for highly charged emotional responses of the patient. The therapist listens, validates, and mirrors the client in a supportive and positive manner.

• ***Suggest structure when the patient is not in session*** such as joining a support group, a self-help group or a community treatment center. Readings such as those listed in Chapter 14, may also be helpful.

• ***Suggest out of session assignments or homework*** to help develop interpersonal skills for the patient and solidify the goals of treatment. For example, suggestions that help the patient strengthen communication with the physician may be helpful. A woman might make a list of questions so that she does not forget to ask them when she feels anxious or hurried. She might select another person to accompany her to the medical consultation, because it can be difficult to absorb the information, and two pairs of ears can be better than one. A number of other suggestions appear in Chapter 2.

• ***Offer a follow-up appointment*** or series of appointments at spaced intervals following termination of treatment for those patients who need continuity.

• ***Suggest alternative modalities of treatment*** such as family, couple or group therapy, if the patient needs further treatment or if the family members also experience a need for help in dealing with the illness.

• ***Offer to extend the number of sessions beyond the initial contract*** if this is necessary for the patient.

• ***Refer the patient for long-term therapy*** if it is clear that short-term methods are not suitable.

■ *BASICS OF THE CRISIS INTERVENTION APPROACH* – Another psychological approach is the Crisis Intervention Approach. This is based on an appreciation of the experiences of the patient during the emergency, one in which she may feel that all of her traditional problem-solving methods have been overwhelmed. As with STDP, the therapist responds situationally and functions actively during the treatment.

■ *EXPERIENCE OF THE PATIENT* – Although the literature (Lazarus, 1983) has shown that the woman will make a cognitive appraisal of the situation and respond according to her assessment of her own internal and external resources, the personal experiences of oncologists suggest that the diagnosis of breast cancer often shatters all of a woman's defenses (Richard Margolese 1991, personal communication). Typical reactions to this life crisis include:

• *Denial* — a sense of THIS IS NOT HAPPENING; MAKE IT NOT HAPPEN!, often with the concomitant "Kill the messenger: This foolish person is making a ridiculous mistake. If I can just eliminate the messenger bearing that mistake, it will all disappear and my life will go on as before."

• *Undoing* — often expressed through the wish to MAKE IT YESTERDAY.

• *Mourning and confusion* — that no matter what else happens, this woman's life will never again be the same as it was before the diagnosis.

■ *RESPONSES OF THE THERAPIST* – At the stages of initial diagnosis and recurrence, the therapist is both an active listener and a source of support.

• *Orientation* — The patient is temporarily overwhelmed by a life situation which overtaxes her problem-solving ability. The goal is not "curing" a neurosis or psychosis but facilitating and enhancing the woman's quality of life and developing a sense of control over this terrifying experience.

• *Urgency* — The person in crisis feels that her problem-solving ability is overwhelmed, and needs an immediate response. She needs to feel that something is being done, changed, or can be changed; there is a need to perceive action and movement.

> ☞ *The patient may feel immobilized; she needs to emerge even from her initial contact with you with some jointly arrived at, clear position on what needs to be addressed or done. This does not necessarily allow for casual history-taking. When a woman has been given a diagnosis of breast cancer, all responses to crisis are magnified; the life-threatening potential creates a very special kind of immediacy. The here and now is the medium. This action orientation will sometimes take the form of a plan, such as an exercise or understanding the patient leaves with, that makes her feel that she has been heard and responded to. She needs to feel that she has a partner in her race against time.*

- *Focus on strengths and empowerment* — Focus not on the client's weaknesses or pathology, but rather on her strengths; help her to regain her own focus on those strengths and use them to rebuild her world. Reinforce a positive outlook or behavior even if the only visible one is her choice to see a therapist. At a time when all of her abilities appear to be disintegrating, help her rediscover strengths and work with these.

- *Flexibility and involvement* — During the crisis, the therapist is often far more actively involved with the client than during traditional therapy. She must do "whatever the client cannot do for herself, and no more." (Parad, 1965) Depending on the individual patient, the therapist may want to be prepared to:

  ... *Be creative* in interventions and skill-building

  ... *Be a resource person* for all kinds of relevant information. Although you do not have to be an expert in every area of breast cancer, some familiarity and a willingness to learn and discuss relevant information is important, from the impact of nutrition, to the best available surgical treatment. Help the patient take charge of the disease by pursuing up-to-date information. Be prepared to refer her to social service agencies that can offer concrete help (see chapter 14).

  ... *Foster self-reliance* in the patient. Be available as a "benign person, an effective ombudsman" (Schneidman, 1985). If your orientation permits, you may, in certain exceptional cases consider facilitating connections yourself, if, and ONLY IF, the patient is unable to do so herself. Caution is advised, since the therapist who is too active may communicate the message that the patient is incapable.

- *Emphasize hope and expectations* — A sense of hopelessness and helplessness is a part of every crisis situation. It is, therefore, important for the therapist to foster a sense of hope, whether it is for survival, health, or living according to one's goals. Hope is a crucial element in the positive outcome of any crisis.

> ☞ "Promise nothing but expect a great deal." Assume that together you will, be able to make some headway in this situation. Be realistic about your own expectations of your own progress as well as the patients. "Headway" may not necessarily prolong life, but it can certainly enhance the quality of life. However, even as you are doing this you must stay in touch with the legitimacy of the patient's distress; avoid an attitude of "There, there, it will pass", which is trivialization. Help the patient reconnect with aspects of herself which she may be overlooking because of the overwhelming presence of the crisis.
>
> (Puryear, 1979)

- *Support* — It is important for the person in crisis to feel that she is not alone. People in crisis are particularly vulnerable and can easily be helped or hindered by responses from their immediate environment. Thus, an often crucial piece of the patient's function at this time comes from the use of a support network, which includes the therapist. During very trying periods, the therapist may need to be available beyond scheduled sessions.

• ***Encourage self reliance*** — Self reliance is a delicate balance to achieve with a patient. By its very nature, the crisis provokes an alteration in equilibrium. The patient must feel connected and supported, yet independent and competent.

> ☞ *The patient is very vulnerable, prone to becoming dependent, hoping to turn the therapist into a "Magic Mommy". This is tempting to the therapist as well. However, it is a poor route to take, because you will almost certainly disappoint the patient (no one can really be a perfect magic mommy!), and it can lead the patient to feeling even worse because of her dependency. Nevertheless, we know that women's psyches thrive on connectedness (Miller, 1976; Gilligan, 1982; Tannen, 1990), and we also know that perceived support is important in a healthy response to cancer. The emphasis must be on achieving a balance between dependency and autonomy and empowering the individual in the face of a potentially overwhelming life situation.*

• ***Normalize, educate, explore alternative approaches*** — Help the patient to understand that she is dealing with an abnormal situation, rather than an abnormality within herself. Ochberg (1991) suggests:
   ... *Education* - share books and articles with the patient.
   ... *Holistic health* - encouraging the patient to explore areas of nutrition, spirituality, humor, etc.
   ... *Alternative treatments*- many cancer patients explore alternative treatments as part of maintaining their own sense of control. Encouraging this, in concert with more traditional medical treatments, can be empowering to the patient.

Chapter 7
SUPPORT GROUPS/GROUP THERAPY

There is strong evidence for the efficacy of group therapy with breast cancer patients (Spiegel, Bloom, Kraemer, & Gottheil, 1989; Lonergan, 1989; Moos, 1977). A professionally led group can provide direction, interpretation, containment, and facilitation of feelings. And, although a group experience may not be appropriate for every patient, at least it should be considered as a possible modality in the patient's treatment plan.

Group therapy has the advantage of helping patients learn and hone interpersonal skills in a realistic environment. Additionally, and often of particular importance for medically ill patients, group therapy provides treatment in an economically viable manner, when compared to the cost of individual psychotherapy. (Spira & Spiegel, 1991)

Curative Mechanisms and Processes

The strengths of a group treatment modality are many in helping to promote patient recovery.

■ *CATHARSIS* – Particularly in the early stages of the group, catharsis, or an opportunity for patients to unburden themselves of strong feelings, can be healing in itself.

■ *HOPE* – The group modality has a unique advantage over individual treatment in that it can instill a sense of hope and empowerment by conveying a sense of universality to patients—a realization that others have been in their situation, can empathize with them, and provide models of coping.

■ *LEARNING* – Observational learning goes on in groups. Members often gain by exposure to multiple role models and they may discover more than one way to solve problems. Group therapy can become an interpersonal learning laboratory, with opportunities for guided practice and problem solving. Naturally this is a particularly powerful modality for helping patients make changes in interpersonal relating. The group can provide feedback about interpersonal style and can illuminate underlying cognitive assumptions that may be interfering with a patient's recovery.

Types of Groups

There are a number of group experiences appropriate for breast cancer patients. At times, the structure of the group may be dictated by outside variables. This is particularly true if the group is formed as part of a medical, hospital, or community service.

Psychologists may need to adapt their usual styles to that of the larger facility and the wishes of the patient.

> ☞ "Several years ago, a woman surgeon in the Philadelphia area requested that I facilitate a group for her patients who had undergone some form of treatment for breast cancer. Initially, a six week group was designed with two-hour sessions scheduled each week. It was found, however, that many women did not want to make even this short term commitment. Their desire to attend over six weeks fluctuated with their physical health and emotional state. We subsequently presented instead one three hour session. It was well attended and enthusiastically received and is now held twice a year, once in the fall and once in the spring."
>
> (Frank, 1992)

Regardless of the type of group, most groups for breast cancer, at least initially, will resemble a support group rather than traditional group therapy. The group is formed to address the psychological difficulties that evolve out of the illness experience *per se*, rather than from intrapsychic difficulties.

■ *THE SINGLE SESSION GROUP* – requires little commitment. Therefore, it is usually less threatening than an ongoing group. Although patients with some major disturbances may need to be ruled out, there is typically little formal screening of patients. Usually, there is some overall structure or tasks, and the purpose is to facilitate the expression of emotions.

> ☞ At Memorial Sloan-Kettering Cancer Center in New York, a one-session inpatient group is offered after completion of the surgical procedures for primary breast cancer (whether lumpectomy or mastectomy). The group is co-led by a social worker and a former patient. The latter serves as a natural focus for the group. This patient-leader has completed surgery and adjuvant treatment and can share her experiences with the group members. Group members are encouraged to verbalize their emotional concerns during this meeting (Rosalind Kleban, 1991, personal communication).
>
> Another single-session group is offered by Frank (1992). Although her group experience is comprised of more structured exercises, the aim is also to foster emotional self expression among the women in the group. The specific exercises of this group, which can be adapted for longer running groups, appears in the Specific Interventions section of this manual.

■ *THE TIME LIMITED GROUP* – typically meets weekly for a specific period of time, such as 12-16 weeks. There may be weekly topics, or the group may be completely unstructured. For example, one 12-week posttreatment group (available at the Post Treatment Center of Memorial Sloan-Kettering Cancer Center) is offered to patients who have completed surgery and all adjuvant treatments. The group is unstructured and the emphasis is on the expression of patients' feelings (Irma Stahl, 1991, personal communication). Instead of a weekly agenda, each particular session generates its own topic of concern. This group serves as a bridge between the breast cancer-hospitalization-treatment experience and a return to family-work-real life normalcy.

Some psychologists may find, at least initially, that a focal point is helpful in generating discussion. Group questions, rather than limiting the discussion, can serve as jumping off points. These questions can stimulate participants to discuss whatever is of most concern to them.

☞ "The therapist attempts to lead the group away from small talk or technical information about cancer or cancer treatments to more personal emotional issues. The therapist can be most beneficial when engaging the group members to be more active in this process, rather than overtly taking control of the group and guiding them directly. Techniques include asking open ended questions of the group or a group member and by referring a personal statement made by one group member to the other group member. This approach helps the group to gain and enhance control over their own lives in the midst of otherwise uncontrollable illness."

(Spira & Spiegel, 1991, p. 20)

■ **THE LONG TERM GROUP** – for patients with breast cancer. The goals of this group are usually determined by the extent of the illness and the desires of the patients.

Distinctions between usual group psychotherapy (initiated due to psychological dysfunction) and supportive-expressive group therapy (initiated due to physiological dysfunction):

Usual Psychotherapy Group	Supportive-Expressive Group
• comes to group due to psychological difficulties	• comes to group because of illness and attempts to cope with illness
• focuses on what is happening here and now	• focus on now and future, inside and outside the group
• no outside contact amongst members	• outside contact amongst members is encouraged
• heterogeneous psychological problems, relatively homogeneous ego strength	• relatively homogeneous psychological problems, heterogeneous ego strengths

(Based on the model of Spiegel and Spira, 1991. A treatment manual for metastatic cancer is available from Spiegel and Spira, as noted in the reference section for this chapter)

- *Supportive-expressive group therapy* is one type of long-term group therapy (Spira & Spiegel, 1991). For the metastatic breast cancer patient, this group can offer a safe and supportive environment to admit and express feelings, to be supported by others and to examine issues that would be difficult without a supportive setting.

The focus of the group stays primarily within the framework of understanding the emotional component of breast cancer treatment, the illness itself, and the development of better support and coping mechanisms for the woman as she progresses through the various stages of her illness. Unlike traditional group therapy, supportive-expressive groups do not attempt to alter basic personality for changes in the future. The accent is on the here and now. This group approach is suited "for those who are seriously ill and may not have a distant future" (Spira & Spiegel, 1991, p. 18).

■ *TRADITIONAL GROUP THERAPY* – For some patients, especially those who have not had a recurrence, the process of dealing with breast cancer may allow them to break through their defenses to do deeper psychological work. These women may be ideal candidates for more traditional group therapy. Here, the emphasis is less on the disease and more on improving overall psychological functioning.

☞ *The difference between a supportive-expressive group and a traditional psychotherapy group is best illustrated by the following example:*

"If a patient states that she feels isolated from her family and from her friends, a common technique in therapy would be to discuss how they are similarly splitting themselves off from the group, and how this pattern plays out in various aspects of their life. By making such unconscious patterns conscious, the patient may be able to recognize this tendency with members inside as well as outside the group, and begin to act in a way which will be more beneficial for them in years to come.

In supportive-expressive therapy for the severely ill, patients may not have years ahead of them in which to implement such a strategy. Instead, when a patient makes a statement that they feel isolated from friends or family, the therapist can re-direct them experientially to others in the group. "Lisa, do you feel comforted by anyone in the group?" Or, "Lisa, are you able to connect with anyone here, now"? Or, "Mary, how do you feel about Lisa feeling isolated? You were just saying how much you enjoyed her in group". Thus, rather than abstracting the concept of Lisa's isolation to reflect upon in order to facilitate long-term change, the group is an opportunity to help ameliorate such feelings of isolation immediately. If this allows for longer-term changes, that is seen as a welcomed additional benefit."

(Spira & Spiegel, 1991, pp. 21-22)

Considerations in Establishing a Group

The following issues will be more or less important depending upon the type of group—single session *vs.* ongoing group therapy. In general, the briefer the time span and the more structured the group, the greater the toleration of heterogeneity among group members. Conversely, when a traditional, ongoing group therapy is planned, more homogeneity on both medical and psychological variables may be desirable.

■ *GROUP COMPOSITION* – An issue to consider in forming a group is patient composition, because group interaction will be a key treatment component. The group leader might consider symptom variables as well as sociological and characterological factors. A good rule of thumb is to strive for a balance between sufficient commonalities so as to promote group cohesion (some of this is provided naturally because this is a content–focused group), but enough variation in membership to provide optimal opportunity to share a variety of perspectives.

• *Similarity of symptoms* — Initially, the leader will have to decide whether the group consists of patients with the same or mixed cancer diagnosis. Will members be patients with an initial, or recurring cancer? The therapist may have control over this decision during the initial formation of the group, and in short-term groups. When a long-term group is planned, there is no foolproof way to predict either metastasis or cure, so the group leader should be prepared to deal with the impact of patients with recurrences on patients who are in remission. It should also be noted that those patients with recurrences may exhibit a preference to be part of a group that has other members who are similarly ill. It may not be helpful to be the only one in the group with a metastasis.

• *Psychological assessment* — More traditional psychological categories, such as character structure and sociological variables can be assessed as well. Consider the patient's personality structure to the extent that it may detract from compliance with medical treatment, and interfere with group process. Other personality issues can be addressed within the group format, such as the capacity for personal assertiveness.
  ... *History-* As a rule, the best predictor of future behavior is past behavior. Assess patient's previous history in group—including roles in family and among peers (school and work).
  ... *Identifying problem patients-* Try to identify potential isolative and potentially destructive members. Excessively needy or angry patients, excessively withdrawn patients, or patients who are sufficiently different from the group so as to be perceived as deviant may be difficult to incorporate into a particular group. Destructive members are at high risk for becoming isolates and, as a result, premature drop-outs. When possible, the addition of individual sessions can provide a bridge to promote connection for these and other decompensating patients. A decision can be made whether to use combined (same therapist) or conjoint (different) therapists. Combining group and individual therapists can be particularly effective in bolstering a fragile patient's sense of connection with the group.

■ **RESISTANCE TO GROUP** – Patients may resist joining group for a variety of reasons. Common sources of resistance include:

• **Shame** — shame about self-revelation.

• **Burdening** — anxiety about being burdened with the troubles of others.

• **Disbelief** — lack of belief that peers can understand and be useful to them.

• **Fear of contagion** — is an additional source of reluctance that can be especially prominent in cancer groups. Patients fear that the emotions shared in group will be invasive and overwhelming. This is an especially common concern when patients are denying, minimizing or intellectualizing about their illness.

• **Staff resistance** — at hospitals may also be a problem. This resistance may be manifested as either failure to refer or as undermining the treatment by interfering with attendance. If you are working within a hospital environment, it is important to develop collegial relationships with hospital staff—including all those with direct patient contact—and to understand the hospital power structure and your place in it. Communicate the purpose of group treatment, and its place in the patient's overall health plan.

General Suggestions for All Groups

■ **OPENING SESSIONS** – The primary goal in working with breast cancer patients is to facilitate open communication with the patient and supporting the development of coping skills. As the facilitator, you can help group members support individual strengths as well as to build the strength of the group. It is important to recognize and respect patient defenses, but it is also important to recognize external reality.

In the opening sessions, verbal participation can be encouraged by modeling a leadership role. Some leaders organize their role by using opening sessions to impart health care information. The leader models participation and respect. The leader also serves as gate-keeper in maintaining group boundaries and encourages the participation of all group members.

■ **FACILITATING THE GROUP PROCESS** – In working with patients who are coping with illness, loss of health, and compromised functioning, it is important to keep basic stages of adaptation in mind as a guideline (although patients do not go through them in linear fashion). Initially, patients confronted with loss may react first with shock and denial, and later, with depression and helplessness. It is important to help patients mobilize the anger and aggression that underlies these other reactions. This aggression is energizing and may be eventually channeled into more effective adaptation. Patients also may utilize grandiosity ("I can do anything") and idealization of caretakers as means of coping. Again, depending on the goal of the group, group leaders can gently challenge these defenses and help patients develop more realistic coping strategies.

Typically, therapists will need to be more directive and active in beginning group sessions, intervening far more frequently than in later stages to move the group from vague external generalities toward more specific emotional expressions.

> ☞ *The therapist might facilitate a group member's initial expression of "People just aren't very nice when they're stressed out, to "Connie was not very nice when she said that to Paula."*
>
> *A similar example would be moving the patient from "I am not very nice when I get stressed out" to "I was not very nice when I talked to my boss at work today."*
>
> *(Spiegel & Spira, 1991)*

As group members become more comfortable with self-expression, therapists can "take a back seat", emerging to provide direction when the group becomes derailed (see later section on managing difficult sessions).

BASIC THERAPIST INTERVENTIONS TO PROMOTE INDIVIDUAL EXPRESSIONS

from	to
External content focus (focus outside of group)	Personal and responsive (focus on self and self in relation to other members)
Abstract (topic is generalized or nebulous e.g. "people say..."	Topic is specific (concrete situation or about a specific person)
Intellectual expression, use of abstract words	Clear and open affect in expression

(adapted from Spiegel and Spira , 1991)

■ **MANAGING COUNTERTRANSFERENCE REACTIONS** – Professional peer support and supervision is often quite helpful for group leaders who are dealing with cancer patients. All kinds of problems occur in a group. Professional consultation should focus upon ways of handling various situations that occur in the group setting. Some issues to be explored are:

- *Fantasies* — Explore leaders' fantasies of the initial group meetings.

- *Prejudices* — Expectations and prejudices regarding cancer patients can be present. It is helpful to articulate these feelings ahead of time.

- *Countertransference* — The reactions of the therapist to the patient must be attended to. A more comprehensive discussion of this issue can be found in the Countertransference section of this manual.

- *Anxieties* — Group leaders may have anxieties concerning whether patients will talk sufficiently and whether the leader will be criticized ("ganged up on") for their inadequacies. Other anxieties may involve fear of depletion by needy patients, or having to live up to an idealized, omnipotent role that feels fraudulent. A new leader may also be anxious about dealing with "bad outcomes" such as recurrence or death.

> ☞ *Training of group therapists for breast cancer patients can be enhanced by the use of a co-therapist, observing other therapy groups, co-leading a group with an experienced therapist, observing video taped sessions, and using a training-treatment manual, as well as ongoing formal group training and supervision.*

■ *MANAGING DIFFICULT GROUP SESSIONS/PROBLEM PATIENTS* – The manner in which the group leader understands and deals with difficult patients and difficulties at the group level depends upon the group contract. If the primary group treatment goal is to support defenses and improve coping in a medically ill patient population, certain situations, such as silence or interpersonal conflict, will be interpreted and handled differently than in a group aimed at personality change. However, in each type of group, it is important to understand the possible meaning of these events, since this influences how one might intervene.

Some of the more trying situations that might emerge in groups are:

- *Frequent absences* — for unknown or unexpected reasons

- *Lengthy silences* — that occur routinely

- *Unproductive norms* — that can perpetuate pervasive depression and hopelessness, or can support unproductive, excessive hostility. Subtle group norms can develop that may be difficult to change such as "Queen for a Day", in which patients compete for who has the most sympathy-arousing situation. Often patients with "lesser" troubles then feel constrained from self-expression, because they feel unworthy of attention.

- *Difficult patients* — may be scapegoated by other members of the group. Difficult patients may attempt to monopolize the group or they may act as help-rejecting complainers.

☞ *Some suggestions for managing difficulties within the group are:*

- *Frequent Absences* - *The psychologist needs to determine whether an absence is due to medical or psychological reasons (e.g., ill health or resistance). It may help to have a group discussion on what kinds of illness, symptoms , or pain could keep members from coming to the group. When a patient is too ill to come to a session, it can help to maintain telephone contact with that patient. In the event of a long absence, develop procedures for reintegrating the member back into the group. For some patients, individual sessions may be helpful before they reenter the group; other patients will not need such a bridge.*

- *Long silences - For the most part, silence will occur less when the therapist is more active and the therapy is structured. Silence can also be counter-acted by having the group become involved in problem solving. As in any group therapy, silence can be considered as resistance. It may be helpful to discuss this in general and externalized areas such as their physician's, spouse's or family's silence, or more directly in terms of the patient's silence in each of these relationships. The therapist may also ask: "If the group was over, and you are at some point in the future looking back, what might you have wished you would have said or done in the group, that you are not saying now?" or "What has been of benefit for you in the group, thus far, and how would you like the group to develop in the future so that you can get what you need from it?" (Spiegel & Spira, 1991)*

- *Problem patients - To work with the scapegoated patient, the group leader might point out the unwanted feeling or symbol the scapegoat evokes for the group. For the help-rejecting complainer, ask the patient to describe what she has done herself, before allowing other patients to offer help. Point out the frustration of the group and encourage the patient to develop alternate ways of relating to the group. To address the "Queen for a Day" syndrome, actively promote a norm which encourages participation from all and be ready to directly talk about this norm, if necessary.*

Chapter 8

SPECIAL POPULATIONS: high-risk women, lesbian women, women of poverty and ethnicity, and older women

This section is intended to alert psychologists to the needs and issues of four special populations of women with breast cancer. Bear in mind that each category is heterogeneous, and the needs of any one particular woman may vary considerably.

High-Risk Women

Women vary in their awareness of their risk status for breast cancer. An alert ear to clinical information presented during intake, or discussion of life events, may offer an opportunity to impart information regarding breast cancer, when appropriate. Although women may have strong emotional reactions to their high-risk status, only 20 percent of the women who develop breast cancer have any known risk factors for the disease. There is no single cause for the development of breast cancer. Current beliefs are that the development of breast cancer is influenced by both genetic and external factors (National Cancer Institute, 1992).

> ☞ *"Some factors are known to increase a woman's chance of getting the disease; these include age (over 50 years), family history of breast cancer (the risk of getting the disease doubles for a woman whose mother or sister had it), and personal history of breast cancer (about 15 percent of women treated for cancer in one breast will get cancer in the other breast).*
>
> *Other risk factors include having the first menstrual period at an early age, having a late menopause, having the first child after the age of 30, and never having had children (each of these conditions means that the body produces the hormone estrogen for many years)..."*
>
> (National Cancer Institute, 1992, pp 3-4)

Psychological Issues in High-Risk Women

Typical responses from women in this high-risk category are:

■ *DENIAL* – For some high-risk women, the psychological trauma of the possibility of breast cancer has been sufficient to trigger what could be life-threatening denial, preventing the woman from routine examination and screening, performing breast self-examination, or even responding to a palpable lump in the breast. Fears of finding positive signs should be explored and confronted. In this manner, a psychologist can assist the woman in developing appropriate self-care techniques.

☞ *The Preventive Medicine Institute of the Strang Clinic of New York offers a National Registry Service for high-risk women. To enroll in the registry, women are asked to complete a family history questionnaire. The clinic will then prepare a diagram of the patient's family tree, along with genetic risk information and surveillance recommendations that fit the family history. Participants are asked to maintain a continuing relationship with the program and provide periodic updates in information.*

■ *TREATMENT OVERUSE* – The psychologist can play an important role with those high-risk women whose overuse of medical services is anxiety-driven. Some women may seek out frequent mammograms in an attempt to calm fears by "doctor-shopping" or accessing mobile mammography units. Women who overuse mammography increase their exposure to radiation that could be harmful. The practitioner can address the underlying issues of fear and vulnerability and assist the woman in developing appropriate health consumer behaviors. Current information suggests that mammograms in postmenopausal women improve early cancer detection and survival but the benefit is less demonstrable in very young women. Clearly, any high-risk women will need a baseline mammogram and should consult closely with her physician as to frequency and timing of followup screens.

■ *ANNIVERSARY REACTIONS* – An anniversary reaction is a change in emotions or behaviors on birthdays, holidays or other personally meaningful occasions. For women whose close relatives (mother, sister, daughter) died of breast cancer, anniversary reactions may occur. These reactions can be particularly intense when the relative was the patient's mother (Royak-Schaler, 1992b). The reemergence of the trauma of loss may create signs of depression and anxiety. Given the patient's status as high-risk, there may also be an intensified focus on one's own vulnerability to the disease.

■ *DATES OF VULNERABILITY TO ANNIVERSARY REACTIONS* – There are several significant dates which may activate an anniversary reaction in the high-risk woman. The psychologist's awareness of these target dates can facilitate increased support during vulnerable periods.

☞ *An anniversary reaction may be triggered when the patient reaches the age at which a relative was diagnosed with breast cancer or died of breast cancer.*

For some women, the anxiety that arises during an anniversary period is focused on their daughter rather than on themselves. Therefore, an anniversary reaction can occur when the patient's daughter reaches the age the patient was when the relative was diagnosed or died of breast cancer.

Prophylactic Mastectomies

A prophylactic mastectomy is the removal of all or almost all of the breast tissue in a non-cancerous breast. At this time, there is no consensus on the advisability of prophylactic mastectomies. It is typically considered an option only when the risk factors are extreme, or the woman is extremely distressed over her high-risk situation and the question of quality of life emerges. Some of the factors considered in the decision for prophylactic mastectomy include an increased likelihood of cancer in the breast, tissue changes in the breast seen as precursors to cancer, or a history of breast cancer prior to menopause in first degree relatives (mother or sister). When a prophylactic mastectomy is done, the patient may have the breast reconstructed either immediately or at a later date.

> ☞ The American Cancer Society has expressed "great concern about prophylactic mastectomies. Only very strong clinical and/or pathological indicators warrant doing this type of 'preventive operation'."
> (American Cancer Society, 1986, p.11)

Women for whom this procedure has been a positive choice emotionally have typically watched multiple members of their family die prematurely of breast cancer. These women also meet many of the high-risk criteria, and often have children whom they feel will grow up without them unless they have this procedure. The combination of these factors can create extreme emotional distress (Royak-Schaler, 1992b). The psychologist may serve a useful role in helping the patient discriminate between brief reaction dysphoria and a more chronic negative affect that seriously interferes with quality of life.

Lesbian Women

Lesbian women with breast cancer may face particular hardships because they face a society and medical establishment that may have little or no understanding of their particular needs and issues. The psychologist should be aware of the societal context within which the lesbian patient finds herself and be sensitive to the impact that breast cancer can have on her life adjustment. These issues should be explored in psychotherapy. The psychologist may consider initiating them if the patient does not. Information on the special needs of this population are available from the American Psychological Association (see reference section).

■ BARRIERS TO TREATMENT

• *Medical community* — Although the lesbian woman may have already established open communication with her primary care physician about her sexual orientation and lifestyle, she may face issues of discrimination as she seeks out specialists for the treatment of breast disease. She may also find herself isolated from loved ones due to restrictive visiting policies, or inability to avail herself of a chosen support person during medical examinations and treatments. She may feel alone and misunderstood in support groups, and alienated from her community.

> ☞ *Homophobia refers to feelings of discomfort around people who are gay. Expressions of homophobia range from mild feelings of discomfort to strongly negative affects that can fuel violence. For the lesbian woman, the many physician and medical personnel contacts involved with breast cancer may elicit a variety of reactions, adding stress to an already stressful situation.*

• *Hospital* — In hospitals, conflicts may arise over "approved visitors" whom the hospital may define as relatives by blood or marriage to the exclusion of the lesbian's partner(s) and chosen family. The decisions regarding whom to admit as visitors will vary from hospital to hospital. In one setting it may only require an explanation to the charge nurse; in another it may require hospital administration approval. Within particularly hostile environments, legal intervention may be necessary.

> ☞ *In order to protect her rights and ensure that loved ones are able to be involved in her care the patient may have to explore legal recourse. A durable power-of-attorney may be helpful for the lesbian patient in assigning the right to make medical decisions. Further information is provided in Chapter 5.*

• *Support groups* — In general, breast cancer support groups are geared toward heterosexual women. For the lesbian patient, the issue of group acceptance may be an actual or a feared problem. The psychologist can help the patient assess the situation, and, if appropriate, can encourage her to discuss this issue with the group leader. The psychologist can aid the patient in locating a lesbian affirmative support group (if possible), or by bringing supportive others into the therapeutic relationship.

■ PSYCHOLOGICAL ISSUES

• *Coming out* — The degree to which the lesbian patient is open about her homosexuality with family, physicians, friends, co-workers, etc. will affect her behavior in dealing with breast cancer. The psychologist should have a good understanding of the patient's own feelings about her sexual orientation and how open she is with others in her life. Only the patient can and should make the decisions about coming out, to whom, and when.

• *Family* — Some lesbian women have never discussed their sexual orientation with family members and may feel increased stress by "being in the closet" as family members become more involved in their lives after a diagnosis of breast cancer.

> ☞ *Relatives may question why a "friend" is so involved in the patient's care and step in assuming their "unmarried" daughter/sister/mother has no significant other in her life. They may be uncomfortable with the lesbian community that rallies round the patient and feel their territory is being invaded. They may "move in" to a living space they assume is not shared or insist that the patient come "home" during her treatment. These and other conflicts may arise and bring into sharp focus the lesbian's internalized anxieties and her fears of discovery by family members.*
>
> *These issues can also add strain to the patient's primary and secondary relationships. When there is a partner, she may feel unacknowledged and betrayed, becoming angry at the patient (particularly if the partner is "out" to her own family).*
>
> *Friends may also resent having to alter their behavior and could potentially lose sight of the patient's need for increased social support.*
>
> *The psychologist can help the patient evaluate her own needs in regards to these separate spheres of her life and develop strategies to enhance relationships by strengthening the communication to those significant in the patient's life.*

• *Potential lovers* — Anxieties over disclosure of breast disease/mastectomy to potential lovers is a common concern of lesbian women. As with heterosexual women, issues of when, where, and how to disclose the issue of breast cancer and fears of potential rejection are present.

• *Self-esteem* — The lesbian patient may encounter negative reactions from the many individuals and systems involved in her treatment. When this occurs, these contacts may serve to reawaken her own internalized feelings of discomfort, thereby threatening her self-esteem.

• *Gender identity issues* — Psychologists should be aware that sexual orientation and gender identity are two separate issues. Lesbian women with breast cancer are just that— lesbians and women. By its very nature — involving a body part linked with femaleness— breast cancer presents issues of gender identity for all women and practitioners should assume this process will be similar for all patients, regardless of sexual orientation. However, some lesbians have repudiated what they see as a male-derived definition of femaleness and may experience ambivalence as they work through the feelings of potential loss of the breast. This issue may come into more intense play if the patient attends a cancer support group whose focus is on appearance and traditional views of femininity.

In contrast, some lesbians will be better able to deal with the potential loss of a breast, because they have already confronted issues regarding their femaleness. In any case, the psychologist can assist the patient in the exploration of her own definitions of her femaleness and affirm her sense of self.

• *Couple issues* — Just as breast cancer has an impact on both partners in a heterosexual relationship, both partners in a lesbian couple are also affected. Many of the issues will be the same and require the same therapeutic skills by the psychologist. However, because the lesbian's partner is also a woman, she may experience her own heightened sense of vulnerability to the disease which can impact both her psychological functioning and the relationship. The partner may need assistance in working through her own fears, so that she does not distance herself from the patient. If appropriate, the therapist might consider offering couple sessions after a diagnosis of breast cancer. The psychologist can communicate an acceptance of the lesbian patient's primary relationship and acknowledge the impact on both women's lives.

Women of Poverty and Ethnicity

The psychologist treating an ethnic woman with breast cancer needs to be sensitive to issues of race and cultural diversity, but should be aware that differences across groups regarding breast cancer appear to be dependent on and influenced by environmental and/ or lifestyle factors, rather than ethnicity alone. Issues such as socioeconomic status, access to affordable, quality health care, diet, social supports, fertility, types of physician interventions, and attitudes regarding breast cancer have all been investigated in research on racial differences in cancer incidence and course (Fox & Stein, 1991; Funch, 1987; Newell & Mills, 1987).

☞ "Experts believe that the disproportionately high rate of cancer death in medically underserved and minority groups is significantly influenced by lifestyle risk factors (for example, diets high in fat) and by lack of access to care, so that early detection, diagnosis, and treatment often are impossible. It is important to emphasize that many of these issues are associated with poverty and the special circumstances posed by poverty-driven lifestyles. Low-income people have a 20% higher incidence of cancer for all sites combined; five year survival rates for low-income women with breast cancer are nine percent lower than those for women in upper-income groups, and low-income black women are three times more likely to be diagnosed as having late stage disease than are their upper-income counterparts."

(National Cancer Institute, 1992, p. 2)

Minority women who are poor are likely to have less prevention information and fewer treatment options than their white counterparts. They tend to be underrepresented in clinical trials, perhaps because they have fewer ways of access to such trials. Mammography utilization, an important component of preventive health care, is lower among black women and Hispanic women than white women.

There is evidence that physicians may treat minority patients differently. "Physicians whose practices comprised 50% or more black and Hispanic patients were less likely to follow mammography guidelines than physicians whose practices comprised 50% or more white patients" (Fox & Stein, 1991).

Women of color tend to be overrepresented in lower socioeconomic levels, and women who are economically disadvantaged have poorer survival from breast cancer. Poor women tend to use hospital emergency rooms for primary care (which deters timely treatment seeking and does not foster consistency of care or follow-up), have diets high in fat (which have been implicated in higher incidence of breast cancer), and have less accurate information about prevention and treatment.

As we have noted, many of the issues the clinician needs to focus on when treating ethnic women are attributable to class rather than race. However, in working with any particular woman, race and ethnicity can be important. A minority woman brings her unique cultural context to the experience of breast cancer, and this context must be explored and made explicit. Important questions to ask involve her own background and the meaning of breast cancer in her family and community. Also the psychologist should understand that racism exists and that women of color must deal with it on a daily basis in their lives. Coping with breast cancer can force the patient to confront racist individuals and systems that she might otherwise avoid. The psychologist's vigilance towards these issues can communicate the added support needed to fortify her in these contacts.

■ BARRIERS TO TREATMENT

- *Socio-economic* — Women who are economically disadvantaged face limitations in access to treatment for breast cancer. The ability to pay determines all too often where one goes, who one can see, and when treatment can be obtained. Because minority women are overrepresented among the poor in this country, the issue of poverty often becomes one of racial inequity.

- *Bureaucratic red tape* — For those who turn to a community agency, city hospital system, or other governmental entity, bureaucratic barriers abound. These systems can be impersonal and rigid, an intimidating combination for women who are already disenfranchised. If a woman is illiterate she will have difficulty with the myriad forms such systems require. If she is inarticulate, she may find the system turning a deaf ear to her needs and concerns. The psychologist can provide the needed advocacy, when appropriate, or assist the patient in gaining access to services to help her negotiate for proper care.

- *Family responsibilities* — Poor women are often heads of households and hold the responsibility not only as the breadwinner, but as the sole child care provider in the family. Being away from work or home for breast cancer treatments can be a threat to the family's equilibrium. These issues need to be addressed practically (through social service aids) as well as psychologically.

■ PSYCHOLOGICAL ISSUES

- *Self-esteem* — The psychologist must be mindful of the debilitating effects of oppression on the sense of self. For minority women, even those who have been able to insulate themselves fairly well from daily discrimination, a diagnosis of breast cancer can mean increased interactions with persons and systems where racism is present. Psychological interventions that acknowledge the existence and negative effects of oppression, and that are designed to increase self-esteem are beneficial.

- *Self care* — Poor women often serve as caretakers to those around them, putting their own needs last. Dealing with breast cancer requires the ability to assertively engage in one's own treatment and clearly articulate one's need. These opposing forces may result in anxiety or guilt and the psychologist can be useful by assisting the patient in a realistic appraisal of her situation and the skills needed to successfully negotiate it. Permission to care for herself and value her own needs are often critical. Yet these behaviors may be at odds with those that are culturally acceptable for some women.

- *Cultural myths* — In any subcultural grouping, misinformation becomes reified through repetition and lack of challenge. Therefore, as with all patients, the psychologist should explore the individual's understanding of breast cancer prevention and treatment. In minority communities there may be harmful myths that need confronting with particular sensitivity. For communities that have felt lied to and betrayed by the majority culture, confrontation of misinformation may be particularly delicate.

☞ *Examples of cultural myths:*

"Don't bother it if it's not bothering you." This belief that a condition which is not painful cannot be harmful can counteract the benefits of early detection and interfere with prompt treatment.

"If cancer hits the air it will spread." Similarly, this myth can interfere with surgical intervention.

The psychologist must appreciate the power of such beliefs and work with the patient to counteract the ignorance on which they are based, while empowering the woman with knowledge.

The risk of breast cancer rises with age, with two thirds of all breast cancers occurring in women over the age of 50. Women age 65 and older are 6 times more likely to have breast cancer than their younger counterparts. However, only one third of women age 50 and over have mammograms on a regular basis. Older women tend to rely on physician referrals for mammography (which may not occur), or be less aware of their necessity than their younger counterparts (Burg, Lane, & Polednak, 1990; Fox & Stein, 1991). Older women with breast cancer also receive fewer diagnostic, therapeutic and support services (Chu, Diehr, Feigl, Glaefke, Begg, Glicksman, & Ford, 1987). While this population is likely to benefit from assistance in daily living activities, particularly within three months of diagnosis of breast cancer (Satariano, Ragheb, Buck, Swanson, & Branch, 1989), they may have the most difficulty in obtaining assistance. Psychologists are in a unique position to assist their older women patients in overcoming common treatment barriers and to address the emotional components of breast cancer in this population.

■ BARRIERS TO TREATMENT

• *Finances* — many older women have limited financial resources. For women 65 and older, Medicare now helps cover the cost of screening mammograms every other year. There may be community agencies also that offer assistance and the clinician may serve as a referral source to these services.

• *Access* — Transportation can be particularly difficult for older women who no longer drive, can no longer depend on a peer group for transportation, and have no family nearby. These patients may need assistance in locating community services that provide transportation or assistance in accessing public transportation. Fears of using these systems or resistance to accepting help from strangers may have to be addressed in therapy.

• *Lack of referrals* — Physicians may not refer older women for screening mammograms. This may be due to the false assumption that older women cannot tolerate aggressive treatment, even if a lump were found. Unfortunately, failure to refer also may reflect our ageist society in which the needs of the elderly are often given less value and attention. The psychologist can help the patient by making her aware of the need for such preventive treatment and by encouraging her to request a referral from her physician.

■ PSYCHOLOGICAL ISSUES

• *Attitudes toward physicians* — For many older women, members of the medical profession are seen as all-knowing experts, whom one does not question. The older female patient may feel intimidated, both as a woman and as a person needing assistance. She may be afraid to ask questions, challenge treatment recommendations, or request second opinions—all of which are abilities that are helpful when dealing with breast cancer. She also may see the physician as a God-like figure who knows best. Therefore, she does not feel the necessity to be fully informed concerning her condition. Confronting outmoded beliefs and strengthening the woman's sense of power in working with the health profession are both useful goals for the clinician.

- *Lack of social support* — Many elderly women lead rather isolated lives. Peers may be deceased, family may be far away, and physical limitations may interfere with activities. For many, depression and anxiety create housebound situations. The psychologist needs to conduct a careful evaluation of the patient's social network and address the emotional issues that interfere with her being actively involved with others in her world. Lack of social skills, fear of rejection, feelings of inadequacy, shame at needing the assistance of others all can be contributing factors to isolation in the elderly. The elderly breast cancer patient particularly needs to address these barriers, so that she can benefit from cancer support groups, and have the support of someone to accompany her to medical examinations and treatments.

- *Sexuality issues* — For many older women, sexuality was often a subject not discussed in polite society. Feelings of shame or discomfort may arise when discussing their breasts with health professionals, and there may be a resistance to breast self-examinations. These same concerns may inhibit open communication with a sexual partner following a diagnosis of breast cancer or following a mastectomy.

- *Denial* — For many older women, breast cancer is the disease they fear most and some take an "I don't want to know" attitude that interferes with acquisition of knowledge regarding prevention and treatment. These women need to know the value of early detection and treatment of breast cancer.

- *Fatalism* — Just as denial may prevent an older woman from engaging in screening activities, fatalism may prevent her from seeking treatment following a diagnosis of breast cancer. For many older women, a diagnosis of cancer is a diagnosis of death. Over the years, they may have experienced multiple cancer-related deaths among loved ones, and remember a time when cancer treatment was not as successful as it is today.
There also may be a belief that with breast cancer, suffering is always present, prolonged, and inevitable, and that the treatment is worse than the disease.

- *Mourning* — For the elderly woman with breast cancer, mourning may be a particularly intense experience. The loss of health has special meaning for the older woman, and she may experience even a treatable breast cancer as the beginning of the end of her life. The deaths of loved ones may also be reactivated for her.

Chapter 9

COUNTERTRANSFERENCE

Countertransference with breast cancer patients raises some specific and unique issues. The therapist is called upon to help a patient deal with a disease over which neither the patient nor the psychologist has control. Breast cancer varies widely in its diagnosis and prognosis. From the start, one must be able to accept that there may be no cure medically or emotionally, and that psychotherapy may be purely supportive. On the other hand, the diagnosis of breast cancer may be medically treatable, and the experience may free the patient to work very actively and productively on major life issues and to experience tremendous emotional growth and change. The psychological response to breast cancer will be influenced by the prognosis of the cancer, the treatment required, the extent of the disability, the social support system, and the premorbid personality of the patient.

Psychologist education about the disease, treatment, prognosis, and typical and atypical emotional responses to the diagnosis, can enable psychological treatment to be more effective. This knowledge can also help the therapist to feel more competent and confident. Therapist gender, age, stage of life, and personal experiences with cancer, loss and illness all have an impact on our interactions with breast cancer patients. Therapist anxiety about disfigurement, physical appearance, sexual attractiveness, and sexual functioning can also be salient factors.

Some of the factors identified as important in the treatment of breast cancer patients may also be relevant to other illnesses or problems. Some, however, will be specific to breast cancer.

Countertransference Issues

■ *MORTALITY* – When dealing with cancer one is faced with the real possibility of a patient's death. The psychologist's feelings about his/her own mortality may surface. This can result in attempts to reduce the fear either by avoidance or by taking an overreactive stance in which one focuses more on the patient's death than is therapeutic for the patient at that stage of the disease.

■ *CONTROL* – Many individuals who are academic achievers develop personalities in which control over their lives has been a motivating factor in their behavior and life choices. Psychologists like to believe that they can positively affect the environment and enable others to experience control over their lives. When the breast cancer patient loses control over her emotions, life, and health, the therapist may be subject to anxiety resulting from loss of control over the patient's future well-being. The psychologist may feel a sense of personal failure if the patient does not recover.

■ *BODY IMAGE* – Breast cancer typically involves surgery, a lumpectomy or the removal of one or both breasts. These procedures can result in disfigurement. The therapist's sense of body integrity and wholeness will be affected by whatever real or imagined visual, tactile, or kinesthetic reactions the patient has to this loss. Breast cancer may involve loss of a body part which is associated with sexuality, femininity, and maternal feelings for women. The male therapist may have difficulty dealing with this particular aspect of the disease with his patient. The female therapist must think about how her own breasts play a role in her identification as a woman, a sexual partner, and a mother. Recognizing one's own beliefs and feelings will enable the therapist to keep from projecting his/her own personal reactions onto the patient.

■ *DEPENDENCY AND HELPLESSNESS* – Any patient with illness, surgical trauma, treatment side effects, and increasing loss of physical ability will be subject to heightened emotional and physical dependency on others. The psychologist's awareness of his or her own unresolved dependency needs and attitudes toward the dependency of others will be important in aiding the patient to deal effectively with her support system as well as the health community. The psychologist may also feel helpless in the face of an incurable illness. It is important to acknowledge this feeling, so that one may move on to areas where one can offer assistance (e.g. you cannot make the cancer go away, but you can help the patient communicate better with the family).

■ *ANXIETY OVER MEDICAL TREATMENT* – Cancer treatment involves high technology. Surgery, chemotherapy, radiation, and bone marrow transplantation all include frightening medical equipment and environments. Being physically invaded by dangerous radiation and toxic drugs are aspects of the treatment a patient may face.

The therapist may want to become familiar with these treatments by visiting the medical facilities. Exposure may reduce the fear and uncertainty that come with having no visual point of reference for the treatments the patient may undergo.

■ *FAMILY HISTORY* – The therapist's own family history of cancer and illness can affect the work with breast cancer patients. The experience of loss from cancer may have an impact on identification with the patient in either a positive or negative manner. If a psychologist has a family history of breast cancer, the process the family member has gone through with the disease will influence the therapist's attitude toward the patient and her prognosis. Recognizing the individual response to a disease and not allowing statistics to overly influence one's reactions to a patient, can greatly enhance the efficacy of psychotherapy.

■ *AGE AND DEVELOPMENTAL LIFE STAGE* – The psychological adjustment to breast cancer is affected by the woman's developmental life stage at the time of diagnosis. The similarity of the therapist to the patient and the current life stage of the patient may create stronger identification with the patient and greater emotional reactivity to the issues with which the patient is struggling. The age of the therapist may foster or limit the patient's comfort level in discussion of the sexual aspects of the disease.

Similarity between therapist and patient might increase therapeutic alliance and the development of empathy, or might create barriers to objective treatment.

■ *DENIAL* – Denial is an important defense for the breast cancer patient. Attempting to process emotional aspects of the disease is an integral part of dealing with a potentially terminal condition. The therapist must be able to respect denial and intervene to confront it only when it is deemed counterproductive to the patient's physical and emotional well-being. Frustration at the slow pace of acceptance by the patient of her prognosis or treatment options will push the therapist into withdrawal or anger toward the patient. Evaluating the degree of denial that is helpful *vs.* counterproductive will be a constant in working with breast cancer patients throughout the course of their disease.

■ *LOSS AND GRIEF* – Sadness and grief over real losses is an integral part of working with cancer patients. Therapists must be comfortable with the patient's sadness as well as their own sadness. It may be appropriate, if the disease enters a terminal phase, for the therapist to share personal feelings with the patient. They may share their feelings of anger at the unfairness of the patient's illness and their sadness about her imminent death. Patients may also appropriately request that the therapist attend the funeral, give a eulogy, or talk with the family. All these departures from traditional therapeutic boundaries take on new meaning when working with a dying or critically ill patient.

■ *SUPERVISION AND SUPPORT* – The therapist working with breast cancer patients will find it helpful to seek the support of other professionals through a formal supervisory relationship, a peer consultation group or other professional channels.

Section IV.

Psychological Interventions with the Family

Chapter 10
HUSBANDS AND SIGNIFICANT OTHERS

Most women in American culture have several relationships of importance which provide psychological support, emotional gratification and practical help. One relationship may be with a husband or long-term partner, and others may be with relatives or friends.

To determine who the significant others are may require some exploration with the breast cancer patient. Whoever is available and willing to help the patient with the multiple needs of her illness must be accepted as the significant other, since in this time of crisis, there is little energy for restructuring existing relationships. Through conversation and questioning, the therapist can help the patient identify significant others in her life. This may be a husband, sister, adult daughter, or a combination of people— for example, one's friends and one's mother. Women may choose to share their emotional experiences with others outside of the family system. A social grid will become apparent, made up of all of the patient's social contacts, and her comparative reliance on each. Friends, extended family, grown children, her own mother, neighbors, and co-workers may all be part of her significant-other network.

Tasks for Significant Others

One way to identify the significant other for the breast cancer patient is to survey the range of tasks that must be handled, concomitant with the illness, and determine how each person, or combination of people, takes care of these needs. In general, the tasks that go with breast cancer include the following:

■ *EMOTIONAL SUPPORT* – Who talks to the patient? Who wants to hear about her feelings and experiences? Who is the person she calls when she has been to the physician? With whom does she feel most at ease, most herself?

■ *TREATMENT DECISIONS* – With whom does she talk over choices? Who does she contact by phone to talk over opinions and reactions? Who is on her side, sees things from her point of view, and with whom she can think?

■ *CARETAKING* – Who are the people who offer concrete help, who change their routines to make time to be with her and help her? Who drives her places? Who helps with the cost of the illness? Since breast cancer is usually a chronic illness, who are the long-term, reliable people who can be counted on after the crisis passes, who help her routinely?

■ *ONGOING FAMILY DEMANDS* – Many women attempt to deny their own needs so that the family will not suffer from an illness. Who helps take care of the everyday chores while she is incapacitated, for example, cooking and laundry? Who makes sure that all of the non-illness daily tasks are done? Most families do not use the many community resources available to help during cancer crises, but, rely on their own supports to get through. Who are the ones who make this happen?

■ *IMPACT ON SIGNIFICANT OTHERS* – Cancer is clearly a crisis for a family, and for the network of people around the patient, regardless of the formal relationship. A great deal depends on the relationships before the illness, with stronger families and friendships faring better than dysfunctional ones.

■ *FAMILY RESPONSES* – During the crisis of breast cancer, some families may deteriorate, and some may improve in their functioning, but most will experience considerable strain as a result of the illness and its consequences. The impact of cancer is so great that it has been suggested that families develop cancer, rather than individuals, and need to be treated as such. Most families respond to the acute phase of the illness, diagnosis and relapse, with a rapid mobilization in support of the patient, followed by a gradual return to routine patterns of life.

> ☞ *In the dysfunctional family, the psychologist may have two separate problems to deal with— the crisis of the illness, and the preexisting problems of the family. When interpersonal relationships are troubled, a woman's need for increased support and security may be problematic. Others around the patient may experience fear of the disease, or fears for their own health, repulsion at treatment or its affects, any of which may lead to rejecting reactions or avoidance of the patient. Others may blame the patient for her illness in an attempt to deal with their own fears or they may reject her increased dependency needs.*

■ *COMMUNICATION PROBLEMS* – Breast cancer patients sometimes describe a "conspiracy of silence" in which family members maintain an attitude of forced cheerfulness, avoiding any discussion of the illness or anything else which might be received as negative. Unfortunately, this isolates the patient with her own feelings, for she is not free to react spontaneously when bound by the same rules of cheerfulness.

> ☞ *The patient may withdraw emotionally, adopting the same attitude and insisting that the illness causes no emotional distress, or she may become increasingly more negative in expressed feelings, in an attempt to establish the legitimacy of her reactions. The more the family attempts to become cheerful, the more negative the patient may become, setting into motion an increasing distance between patient and family members. It helps to get family members to DO helpful things for the patient and themselves, rather than to try to FEEL cheerful.*

■ *MARITAL RELATIONSHIPS* – Relatively few marriages (7 %) end in divorce after a diagnosis of breast cancer (Lichtman, 1982). Sometimes even bad marriages rally, as husbands make special efforts, out of honor, guilt or epiphany, to help wives who are ill. Among divorcing breast cancer patients, it is typically the wife's decision to end a dysfunctional marriage because of the marital strain, which she feels has implications for her health.

> ☞ *In all marriages, a diagnosis of breast cancer causes a good deal of difficulty and disruption for both spouses. In most marriages, women offer more supportive behavior and comments to their husbands than their husbands do to them, although this disparity may temporarily disappear during the initial crisis. Husbands are more apt to be supportive if they attribute the difficulties of the period to the illness rather than to their wives' personality and character. The more information a spouse is given about the disease and its treatment, the more supportive he is likely to be, and the more helpful in the decisions which must be made. Where there is little spousal support, the adjustment of the patient to the illness is generally poorer.*
>
> *Usually, younger couples experience more stress with a breast cancer diagnosis, not only because they are more likely to have young children to care for, but because they have not developed the integrated couple patterns more common to older marriages. Sometimes couples cope with the strain by idealizing each other, so that the others' behavior is seen as "so wonderful," and all reactions are seen as indications of great courage, commitment, and devotion, as well as character and tenacity. This form of stereotyping can, in fact, be quite functional, as the expectations often produce the behavior, as well as enhancing everybody's self esteem.*
>
> *It is difficult for couples to accept the inherent imbalances in the dyad with one sick member. Both members have great pressures, but they are different ones, and both are apt to feel quite needy. A woman may feel a much greater need to discuss her experiences and her feelings, while her husband may react differently. A woman may project internal conflicts onto those around her so that disagreements develop where there is no clear basis for them. Problems in communication are highlighted during the breast cancer crisis so a wife may complain that her husband doesn't really care about her, rather than expressing her specific disappointment at his limited affection and her own self doubts. The husband may be confused by the vague, blameful communication, and may withdraw further, thus strengthening the disharmony.*
>
> *(Vinokur & Kaplan, 1990)*

■ *HUSBANDS AND LONG-TERM PARTNERS* – Initially, the psychologist should assess the marriage (or long-term relationship), its history of problems and disruptions, as well as the existing stresses at the time of diagnosis. For some patients, an offering to include the partner in the treatment plan will strengthen the partnership and enhance relationship skills. In cases where the relationship is peripheral to the patient's life, and she is comfortable with her partner's limited status, it may be best to offer to draw on other caregivers for help in the psychological treatment.

• **Stresses to men** — Men typically experience difficulty when their wives develop breast cancer which is, in part, culturally induced. A woman is apt to be the sole confidant of a man, and her illness changes this relationship. Men encounter serious problems in these circumstances so often that they are frequently considered to be secondary patients.

☞ *The following are some common emotional reactions of men when their partner has breast cancer:*

Emotional Isolation: Because many men tend to rely on marriage for the majority of their emotional and social needs, emotional isolation is a serious problem for men when their partners develop breast cancer. Men may experience physical symptoms, such as those of anxiety, attentional deficit, sleep disorder or fatigue as a reaction to this emotional isolation.

Role Reversal: A husband may be forced to take on the role of wife as well as husband, with disruptions in the normal tempo of his life. He may feel inadequate, angry, or overwhelmed at the new household responsibilities and caregiving for a sick wife.

Emotional Unresponsiveness: The husband may feel unable to deal with his wife's emotional reactions. He may seek professional help for the wife because he feels he cannot be helpful. It is particularly important for the professional in this context to reintegrate the man into his husband role, by helping him to develop some level of useful response to his needy wife. This will help avoid the isolation which can develop in a marriage when a wife is "turned over" to the psychologist for help with her feelings.

Communication Style: The husband may expect his wife to react in the same way that he does. He may compartmentalize his reactions, dealing only with his feelings at certain limited times, and he may expect her to do the same. He may for example, change the subject of conversation, encourage her to smile, and expect her to control her own fears as he controls his, i.e., by repression. She may experience this as a trivialization of her illness. The husband may also be frightened that negative thoughts made her sick, and that fears, anxiety or thinking about cancer at all will cause a recurrence or spread. He may want his wife to make a rapid adjustment to the illness, not allowing her to progress at her own pace.

Death Fantasies: The demands and disruptions of breast cancer are unpleasant, and a husband may have difficulty with resentment and anger at his changed life circumstance. He may at times wish that the problem would end, if not in cure, then in his wife's death. These feelings are common to caregivers in a chronic illness. However, if the man has not had a great deal of experience in exploring and accepting his own feelings, he may be particularly uncomfortable with these reactions. In trying to deny them, they may become more persistent, draining his emotional energy, sapping his self-esteem, and solidifying his repression.

(Lichtman & Taylor, 1986)

■ *IMPACT ON CHILDREN* – The age and needs of dependent children greatly affect the psychological setting for the patient, because they can increase the demand of family energy and time. (A more detailed account of the child's experience appears in the next chapter of the Manual).

• *Very young children* need extensive care and may require the participation of extended family members or the addition of hired help (housekeepers or babysitters) to the family constellation.

• *Adolescent children,* although more self-sufficient, may present a greater challenge, because of their emotional neediness. They may seize opportunistically the chance to avoid parental supervision that an illness provides, or they may resist the demands to give more help and caring at home. Adolescent daughters may present special difficulties to the woman with breast cancer, since the normal stresses of this age are combined with the family's greater need for help, sensitivity and traditional female role behavior. Identification with the mother and worry that "it can happen to me" may also be concerns that may or may not be verbalized.

• *Young adult* offspring may offer the least support to the breast cancer patient, because they are likely to react to her illness by becoming excessively fearful or avoidant. Young adults are typically involved with their own lives and may have little time or energy to give to this crisis situation.

■ *FRIENDS* – Of special importance to women are those networks of friends that offer emotional support and practical help. Friends can offer help in a variety of concrete ways, such as cooking, child care, shopping, transportation, or companionship during medical treatment. There are relatively few complexities to offering help in these ways. Upon diagnosis of breast cancer, most women quickly become aware of the helping people in their lives, and may choose to encourage these relationships, letting other relationships fade. The exposure to new people in medical settings may prompt the development of new, illness-inspired friendships which may endure.

> ☞ *The strengthening and emergence of new relationships is important, as survival correlates with cooperative, mutually satisfying relationships for the breast cancer patient. Often, a woman will feel more comfortable and less constrained in these relationships, allowing more self-disclosure and open expression of feelings. This experience can improve her mood and increase her self-esteem and sense of efficacy.*
>
> *The absence of a network of friendships is considerably more difficult, because it is usually too taxing to try to create these on demand when a woman becomes ill. It is also important to consider why such a network does not exist, and whether this is a reflection of a woman's personality, perhaps alienating those around her, or her unwillingness to help others.*

• *Stress to friends* — Helping a patient with her feelings about the experience of breast cancer requires sensitivity. Giving advice, or encouraging recovery can be experienced as presumptuous and pressuring. Identifying with a patient's feelings by way of offering sympathy, e.g., "I know exactly how you feel," can be experienced as alienating and belittling, because it ignores the patient's unique phenomenological experience, and closes off further discussion. Knowing "what to say" and "saying the right thing" are cause for concern among friends. Expression of caring and interest, along with a readiness to be helpful, are typically the most helpful responses.

☞ *Guidelines that can be offered to significant others when visiting patients:*

Ask before going. A surprise visit is not always welcome. Calling ahead gives the patient a chance to look and feel her best and to schedule visits so they won't interfere with medical care.

When arriving, knock and wait for a greeting before entering the room.

Be prepared to see medical equipment, tubes, bottles, etc.

Greet the person as you normally would (shake hands or kiss)

Find a chair and sit down near the patient. Proximity and eye contact help make the patient comfortable. Do not hover.

Do not compare the patient's present condition to previous states of health. Instead of asking "How are you?" ask "How are you today?" or "How is the day going?"

Let the patient lead the conversation. Be a good listener and don't be unnerved by lulls in the conversation. You need not feel you have to say something.

Visit with a distraction in reserve, ie. carry along recent photographs, a book of short stories or anecdotes, or other items to share if the patient wishes to be entertained.

Remember that patients do not want to think about their illness all the time. It is human to want to laugh and ignore the most serious realities for brief periods. Sports, fashion, politics, music or news about mutual friends may be welcome.

Ask "What can I get you?" or "How can I help?"

If the patient can walk or sit in a wheelchair, suggest a trip around the floor, to the lounge or recreation area or to the gift shop.

Give the patient realistic support or reassurance. You may want to urge the patient to utilize hospital social workers, support services, or chaplains.

It may be helpful to take breaks by going to get something to eat, checking the parking meter, running an errand, etc.

Knowing when to leave is important. For some patients ten minutes is a long time, for others an hour is too short. Say, "I think I've been here long enough." If the patient requests you to stay, you can stay a while longer. If the patient agrees or says nothing, it is probably time to leave.

(adapted from Rowland, 1990, p. 68)

Chapter 11
HELPING THE CHILDREN

Mothers with breast cancer are often vitally concerned with the effect the illness will have on their children. In addition to struggling with their own physical and emotional distress, they must cope with the fears, fantasies, reactions, and developmental needs of the children. The psychologist can be helpful to the breast cancer patient by bridging the disruption of family patterns with strategies to meet the psychological needs of the children.

The overall goal of the psychologist is to "dehydrate and rehydrate"; that is, to diminish the parent's helpless/doomed/overwhelmed states and to provide a helpful framework for the parent to use with a child. It is important to avoid burdening the parent, however. Just as we would not want the parent to overload a child, we would not want to overload the parent.

Our society places value on protecting children from insecurity and the idea that human beings are mortal. In the face of a potentially life-threatening illness in the family, we still want to protect them to the degree possible; but to the degree that it is not possible, the uncertainty of life must be faced at the appropriate time.

Strategies

The following highlights some of the important dimensions to help children cope.

■ MAKE THE ILLNESS MANAGEABLE FOR THE CHILD

• *Break the news to a child a little at a time* — The parent can give a realistic and limited picture, not a tragic projection. The message should convey that the illness has been discovered, treatment is occurring, and the family is in the situation together. If the mother is able to handle her own emotions, she is the best person to to tell the child. If she is unable to do so, whoever will be substituting as primary caretaker for the child may act for the mother.

• *Give information to the child according to the child's capacity to integrate it* — The message is one of a mother who loses a breast for the positive purpose of saving the whole body. One may communicate with dolls or toys to a young child, with song or story to an older child, with straightforward non-alarmist language to an adolescent.

• *Don't see through the defenses of a child too quickly* — Some children may need to hold the news at a distance, as if the story were happening to someone else. The child may need to sublimate, to obtain needed catharsis through alternate channels. Some may need to return later and hear the explanation all over again. Other children may show little or no initial reaction, which can be unsettling to parents. Some children may have insensitive reactions, which seem selfish and may anger or hurt the parents' feelings. Children need time to assimilate such important news.

• *Support the child's partializations and emotional resolutions* as well as letting the child know about the adult activities and solutions that are working. Children often have their own answers to very difficult questions, which we need to hear and respect as in the classic revision of Thurber's (1990) story of *The Princess and the Moon,* wherein the little Princess devises a way to possess the moon.

■ *MAINTAIN CONTINUITY*

• *Keep the child's routine and predictable world in order* — as much as possible, and even expand outreaching opportunities if possible. It is a powerful message for a child to feel the world is *not* ending, but is continuing to grow and be enriched.

• *Predict and communicate the absences of the mother* — whenever she must be away from home for hospitalization or treatment. Partial restitution for loss and strain may be offered for the young child by leaving a photograph or by leaving little presents to be opened each day, at a time when mother and child would usually spend time together. For the school-age child, affectionate postcards or tape-recorded messages can be prepared before the mother leaves and later delivered to the child at intervals during her absence. If phone calls and/or visits are possible, the direct contact can be even more reassuring. However, care may have to be exercised in exposing the child to the treatment setting.

■ *ALLOW FOR INDIVIDUAL REACTIONS* – Probably the most salient influence on the child's reactions is the parents' manner of reacting and coping. The particular way a child responds will depend on age, temperamental style, the course of the mother's illness, the degree of change in the family's life, and the availability of support for the child.

Typically, it is the very young child who has the greatest difficulty with being separated from the mother, although at any age a child may regress to earlier stages of their lives. If the mother's illness is protracted, the responses and needs of children will change as they mature developmentally.

The psychologist can help the parent recognize the child's coping style and receive the messages being conveyed. Helping the parent to listen can facilitate appropriate offers of support, acceptance, reasurrance, or assistance, including outside professional help when necessary. Often, children derive great benefit from participating in a support group of peers, whose parents are also cancer patients.

☞ *Identifying a child's problematic reactions enables the parents and/or the psychologist to ease distress and foster continuing development. Samples of likely problems which can occur at different age levels in children whose mothers have breast cancer follows. (Note: A caveat of caution—All children have problems. Loving adults and concerned psychotherapists can, at times, be excessively vigilant and incorrectly ascribe the etiology of all aberrant behaviors to the breast cancer experience):*

Pre-school children
- *Separation anxiety, which may be exacerbated by the mother's own anxiety in leaving for treatment and being parted from a very young child.*
- *Depressive reactions due to mother's incapacity and unavailability, which may be perceived as lack of love and interest.*
- *Resistance or overattachment to new caretakers.*
- *Rejection of mother, because of her absences or physical changes such as bandages, new body odors, etc.*
- *Odd or magical fantasies about the cause of the household disruption.*
- *Anger at the changes in routine and relationship patterns.*

Latency age children
- *Helplessness, and perhaps eventual depression, when the need for mastery is thwarted by the powerful family crisis.*
- *Guilt and anxiety at "bad thoughts" as a betrayal of mother, an impediment, or even destructive of her.*
- *Emotional isolation due to difficulty in verbalizing feelings or in finding adults to listen.*
- *Embarrassment at the attention that the mother's illness draws.*
- *Fears for their own health based on misunderstanding about contagion or inheritance.*
- *Difficulties in dealing with doctors, nurses, hospital rules, or machines.*

Pre-adolescence and adolescence
- *Power struggles, anger, guilt, and feelings of abandonment may result from changes in supervision that leave the child either too little guidance or overcontrolled.*
- *Sense of infringement or unfair burden, due to the addition of new responsibilities for chores and sibling care.*
- *Changes in family dominance patterns due to the mother's incapacity may leave teens in a new role with father and siblings. This may be particularly uncomfortable for girls if they take the mother's former role. When the mother recovers, the return to normal may also present problems.*
- *Embarrassment at sexual associations to the breast.*
- *Discomfort with the increasing focus on the parent, when the teen is striving for more distance and autonomy.*
- *Anger at the inconvenience or disruption of social activities. This is particularly pronounced when the teen must rely on the parents for transportation.*
- *Anger at reduced financial resources and support.*
- *Loneliness or sense of being an outsider if friends withdraw due to their*

(continued on next page)

☞ *discomfort with the illness or the changed routines.*
- *Preoccupation with their own physical appearance and possible rejection of mother because of her changed appearance.*
- *Uncertainty about the future, especially if the mother is single.*

Young adult
- *Resistance against the threat to newly developing independence from the family.*
- *Overattachment and difficulty with separation of identity and development.*
- *Guilt about neglecting the parent in need.*
- *Denial, in the form of minimizing or forced cheerfulness, and the refusal to acknowledge mother as a suffering adult.*

■ BALANCE BETWEEN FOCUS AND DISTRACTION

• ***Children show a wide range in their capacity and their need to know what is happening to the mother's body*** — Be sensitive about a child's wish, fear or readiness to see any wounds, as well as the mother's wish, dread or readiness. Factors such as the child's age and the usual family practices around nudity, bodily functions, and illness must be considered. It is important to protect the child from experiences that will be overwhelming and frightening. On the other hand, a family may believe that it is important to honor the right to know what has happened and not create a taboo. Whether or not the child sees the surgical site, the aim is to put the wound in perspective with the goal of a healthy body for the future.

• ***Distract the child from an unremitting focus on the mother's status, when feasible and appropriate*** — A new horizon serves to point the child toward individuation and greater independence. To the extent that a child can develop a focus outside the mother, that process will aid in individuation. This, in turn, will increase the child's ability to cope with the mother's illness.

■ ACKNOWLEDGE THE INTERSUBJECTIVITY

■ ***ACKNOWLEDGE THE INTERSUBJECTIVITY*** – Both mother and child are experiencing something important. Because of the magnitude of the mother's drama and her need for support, it may be even more difficult for her to support the experience of the child. The inner resources of both are strained. If there is a father or significant other in the household, his experiences are also important, and his intrapsychic and interpersonal style of handling emotions and the vicissitudes of the illness contribute to the child's experience. Similarly, the experiences of siblings add to the interplay within the family matrix.

• ***When parents react to the mother's cancer as if it is a tragedy for the child, then it is*** — It is important for parents to know what "tune" they play to the child for the child to play back.

• *Parents are in a contradictory dilemma* — How do they share, support, and communicate with a child, but not pour their own feelings into the child? One of the hardest emotional tasks is for the mother to bear the responsibility for her own tragedy and not exploit the child as an instrument of expression. The mother cannot look to the child to be herself. For example, when the mother is sad, she must experience her own sadness and not project it to the child. Children have their own sadness, anger, anxiety or other feelings. It is helpful to remember that children often do not respond as adults expect them to.

In some instances, the psychologist may work directly with the child and his/her internal world of intersubjective relations. The goal is to tap the inner objects and representations that can be good and be maintained for the child. Sometimes the inner representations of a relationship can be modified toward a more mature stance.

• *The child's omnipotent fantasies must be recognized* — After all, a child often wants and needs to believe the parents are superpowers. When a parent proves vulnerable, the child may seek magical strength within. The child may imagine that the mother's illness is his or her fault. The child is then burdened with having to be extraordinarily good, sweet, and undemanding to try to remedy the situation. The parents and others in the support network must reassure the child that cancer is not his or her fault. Neither is it the parents' fault; certainly they are not omnipotent, either, despite the child's wish that they could be so. When the mother is ill, the child's need for idealization, strength, mirroring, oneness may be partially achieved through relationships with others, such as the father, other relatives, or the psychologist.

Affective States

From toddlerhood on, the children of a woman with breast cancer need the emotional latitude to have their own feelings in response to the illness, to express them as they are capable, to share them with someone who is trustworthy, and to have their feelings respected. Their greatest challenge is both to handle and to work through these feelings and contain them within manageable limits.

A child may act staunch or may act clingy or may vacillate between the two reactions. A child may cry frequently or play the comedian. A child may act sullen and withdrawn one day and empathic and caring the next day. Almost every child will feel frightened, confused, sad, self-pitying, or guilty at some point. The expression of these feelings will vary considerably. However, some children will react overtly only to daily events and not to the impact of the overall illness. Prepare the child who is old enough to understand to expect conflicting feelings, e.g. that it is normal both to love and to feel resentful of the ill parent.

■ *ANXIETY* – The child of a mother with breast cancer is usually anxious, although some children will mobilize extreme denial and will not appear anxious at all. Such a child is full of "what ifs?" which the parent must answer and address in a partial way that is sufficient to ease the child's worry. The child may be anxious about what will happen to himself or herself, to the mother, to the father, and to other family members, even the pets. He or she may become anxious also about such concerns as how to meet the extra demands to perform and contribute, or about how to respond to the family's increased financial burden. Overall, the child is anxious about the changes and the unknown and uncertain future.

- *To reduce anxiety* — ensure that the child has multiple sources of information and support available. When the child can talk with a physician, see a film, read a booklet, join a group, as well as discuss matters with family, it can be reassuring. In addition, the access to outside resources works to counteract secretiveness, which is anxiety-provoking in and of itself. In a single-parent household, it is especially important for both the mother and the child's well-being to enlist additional sources.

- *Coach the child* — who needs help in what to say to the mother or to others, what to bring as a gift to the hospital, or what tasks might be performed to make a contribution. It seems that adolescents especially tend to flee or pretend nothing is happening. They may fear doing something wrong. Perhaps even more than the younger child, they need direction to know their place and be given the opportunity to claim it, yet they often find it hard to ask for guidance.

- *Prepare for the moment* — when or if the child asks if mother will die. At this point the child needs reassurance that is believable. A parent might say "Everyone dies eventually, but right now mother is getting good treatment to help her get well and the physician knows what he or she is doing." Leave hope in any response to the child and communicate that the whole family is trying its best and are working together.

■ *ANGER* – Anger is a natural response to frustration, pain, and loss. It is to be expected that on occasion a child will become angry at the parent for being ill, at any authority figure who must ask the child to do more and receive less, at playmates or siblings (who are handy targets), at God, fate or the inchoate universe because someone must be to blame for such a terrible set of circumstances.

In general, if the anger can be vented, not left to simmer, and if the child's pressing needs at the time can be sensitively addressed, the anger will subside. It is essential to reassure children that the ill parent will not be destroyed by their anger. To the contrary, sometimes their anger can join with the anger of the mother and be channeled into a positive fighting spirit. Sometimes the anger must be lived through, because there is no ready relief for the time being.

Guilt is often a by-product of anger. The child may feel quite remorseful for feeling selfish, greedy, resentful, out of control, and for lashing out or complaining. In that case, they need help to make appropriate amends (such as picking up the items they have hurled to the floor and saying a simple "I'm sorry," when they mean it) and forgive themselves as well as accept forgiveness.

■ *GRIEF* – Sadness, helplessness and regression accompany significant loss and the threat of further loss — both mother and child will experience these states to some degree. Psychotherapy can help the mother so that her helplessness and regression do not traumatize the child. Psychotherapy supports the parent to better share the active doing and coping with the child, rather than only the depressive elements. Nevertheless, sadness and grief are natural responses and will be part of the family's landscape also. No one can eliminate the child's grief, but it can be shared so that the child does not have to face it alone.

During the mournful time when a mother is experiencing great loss in the terminal phase of the illness, the child has a special need too — the child is struggling to maintain and remember the courageous, alive, vital mother. The child can find courage in the knowledge that if mother can face this loss, then he or she can too. Life can be borne.

Section V.

Interventions and Resources

Chapter 12
SPECIFIC INTERVENTIONS

When the patient is newly diagnosed with breast cancer, or is in a crisis of recurrence, it is usually advisable for the therapist to take an active and supportive stance. For some patients (and some psychologists) specific exercises may be useful during this stage of treatment. The value and appropriateness of such interventions have to be determined by assessing the skills and therapeutic style of the psychologist in concert with the needs of the individual patient. Clearly, these techniques are not for everyone. The more traditional psychologist, operating in an active, supportive and empathetic manner, may be as effective as the less traditional psychologist. The following suggestions are offered as possibilities for enhancing treatment effectiveness.

Existential-Humanistic Techniques

Some of these exercises come from the Bioenergetic (Lowen, 1977; Pierrakos, 1977) orientation. The primary thrust of this work is that many of the significant things that happened to us in our life were experienced pre-verbally, before we had language. The theory is that areas of affect are located within the body and can be expressed non-verbally, through "body work." This can be beneficial to breast cancer patients by teaching them to "tune in" to the area of their body in which they experience stress, anger or tension. This way, we can help them use that area as an "early warning sign" of growing discomfort, and help target that area for appropriate release.

> ☞ *The therapist should bear in mind how vulnerable an individual is in crisis. They may easily abdicate their power to you and allow you to lead them into exercises that would ordinarily be unacceptable to them. The therapist needs to use good judgment in deciding the relevant effectiveness of the exercise with any client. The client's own self-respect should never be compromised. One way to overcome this is to have the therapist do the exercise alongside of the client. This helps to overcome the client's resistance and feelings of discomfort.*

■ BASIC ANXIETY-REDUCING EXERCISES

• *Focused breathing* — Essential to all attempts to help an individual calm herself is the use of a most powerful tool within each of us: our breathing. If the patient can become aware of how to use breathing effectively, she has the ability to change her stress level within herself at all times. Since a crisis situation aggravates the stress level, any client in crisis can benefit from the simple awareness of her breathing.

These exercises can be done individually or in groups, with or without a therapist present, standing up or lying down.

> ☞ *Become aware of your breath. Breathe comfortably and easily, and imagine your breath as a peaceful presence that enters your body to bring it peace. Direct your breath to a place below your navel, what the Yoga people call the "Hara." Imagine your breath going down to that place and calming all of the body as it does this. Then become aware of any part of your body that is tense. Bring your breath to that muscle or area and become aware of how much more relaxed it can become as your breath touches it. Now place your hand on the spot below your abdomen where you are directing your breath. Feel your arm becoming more and more relaxed as you do this. Continue for as long as you need to feel your body relaxing.*

• *Centering* — This exercise is almost as portable as the breathing exercise. It gives the participant a renewed sense of power and control over her life, two of the most essential issues in crisis intervention.

> ☞ *Stand with your feet about ten inches apart, knees bent in what skiers call the "snowplow" position. Keeping your knees bent, allow your body to fall forward until your head is hanging down as close as possible to your feet. Breathe deeply. Using your fingertips to maintain your balance, and keeping your knees bent, slowly raise your heels off the ground. Experience the vibrations that go through your legs and into your body as you do this. Stay this way for as long as you can, and then slowly return your heels to the ground, keeping your knees bent. Slowly raise your upper body to an upright position and then raise your arms above your head. Explore the space around you and become aware of the space you own in the world. As you do this, stay in touch with your own inner center, and say out loud if possible, "I'm alive!"*

• *Progressive relaxation* — This is basically the traditional Jacobsen approach (see Simonton et al., 1980, for further examples). *See pointer box page 95*

Anger Expressive Exercises

There are some anecdotal data that link difficulty in expression of anger with cancer formation, but it is not conclusive by any means. Neverthless, as clinicians we know that the experience of breast cancer involves numerous life changes including interactions with the medical system and confrontations with mortality. These experiences can generate frustration and anger which, when expressed in a safe, protected environment, can be an experience in empowerment, one which our culture often denies to women.

• *Hitting* — The following is derived from Lowen (1977) and is best done in an individual session. *See pointer box page 96*

☞ *A typical progressive relaxation exercise would be:*

Lie down in a comfortable place. Breathe easily and regularly. Focus on your breathing. As you inhale, feel your breath bring peace and calm to every part of your body. Do this for a few minutes.

At your next inhalation, point your toes and stretch the bottoms of your feet. Hold your breath, and as you do so, hold your feet in the outstretched position. Then gently exhale and relax your feet. Breathe comfortably for a few minutes.

At your next inhalation, tighten your leg muscles and stretch your legs. Hold this position as you hold your breath, then gently exhale and relax your legs. Breath comfortably for a few minutes.

Feel your legs becoming warm, heavy and relaxed.

When you next inhale, tighten the muscles of your buttocks; hold this tightness as you hold your breath. Gently exhale and relax your buttocks. Breathe comfortably for a few minutes, then inhale and tighten your stomach muscles; hold this tightness as your hold your breath. Gently exhale and relax.

Feel your whole lower half of your body becoming heavy, warm and relaxed.

Inhale, and make your hands into two fists and pull your arms straight down, as if you were pulling them out of their sockets. Hold your breath and hold your hands and arms in this tight position, then gently exhale and relax your arms and hands. Breathe comfortably for a few minutes, then inhale and pull your head down and touch your chest with your chin. Hold this position as you hold your breath, for as long as your can. Breathe comfortably for a few minutes, then exhale and relax your head and your chest muscles. Now your whole body is feeling warm, heavy and relaxed.

Breathe comfortably for a few minutes, and when you next inhale, raise your shoulders up to your ears and hold them there as you hold your breath, for as long as you can. Then exhale and relax your head and neck.

Breathe comfortably for a few minutes, then inhale and scrunch your face up and tighten all of your facial muscles. Become aware of how much tension you are carrying on your face and tighten all of those areas. Hold this position as you hold your breath, for as long as you can, and as you exhale relax your face muscles and feel all of the tightness dissolve.

Now breathe comfortably for a while. If there is any part of your body that still feels tense, visualize your breath as a ray of soft warmth that can be directed to that tight place to relax it and heal it. Stay in this position as long as you wish.

Think of a code word for the way you feel when you are relaxed so that you can return to this position any time you need to. Practice saying your code word and feeling your whole body relaxed, warm and heavy as it is now.

> ☞ *Have patient stand or kneel down in front of a bed or soft couch with her arms raised above her head and her hands in fists. Then have her hit the bed with both arms simultaneously, preferably using the whole forearm to hit the bed. This can be done without words or with any kind of language that the patient or therapist finds appropriate to the situation.*
>
> *A variation on this exercise is to use a tennis racket instead of the fists. If standing, the patient's knees should be bent and movement should come from the entire upper body.*

- *Off my back* — This exercise taps another body area for release of anger.

> ☞ *Have patient stand with her feet about ten inches apart and knees slightly bent. Make two fists, bend elbows so arms with clenched fists are in front of chest. Extend lower jaw. Breathe deeply. As patient says "Off my back" out loud, she will pull her arms behind her very strongly until elbows pass behind rib cage. Repeat several times. Encourage voice to become louder and louder.*

- *Kicking* — This exercise can be done either by encouraging patient to stand up and stamp their feet or to kick a safe object (e.g., bean bag) or by lying down on bed and kicking the legs.

> ☞ *Some words that can be used at this time are:*
> *No, no, no (etc)*
> *Why? why? why?*
> *I hate_____*
> *I will not_____*
>
> *Note: If the patient is unable to articulate during this exercise, you may want to help her by suggesting words from her session.*

Visualizations

Visualization is the process of creating visual images and focusing on them in the philosophy of Virgil that "mind moves matter." Visual imagery, in conjunction with medical treatment, improves aspects of the patient's quality of life and may have some impact on longevity among cancer patients. Here, for example, is one visualization (Other examples can be found in Simonton et al., 1980).

☞ *Close your eyes and breathe comfortably. Take yourself to a wonderfully peaceful place: the sun is shining, the sounds of the wind chimes play in the background and songbirds fill the air with their sounds of joy. The sun shines down upon your body and brings with it the sense of hope. As the sun touches your body it creates the beginning of a new you. See and feel the sunbeams touching your body, and visualize a new you slowly and gracefully emerging from yourself, bathed in the warm caresses of the sun. The new you is you at your best; she is strong, healthy and whole, she is beautiful in her body and her spirit. She feels competent and powerful. She is peaceful and relaxed.*

Keep this image of the new you before your eyes. Watch her as she moves about in the sunlight, moving gracefully in the breeze, doing anything she needs or wants to do. Enjoy this you. Keep her image as you do this visualization and take her image with you after you finish, so that you can always see her and recharge your sense of hope in yourself and in your life.

Cognitive-Behavioral Interventions

Both brief cognitive-behavioral interventions (Edgar & Rosberger, 1992) and long-term cognitive interventions (Golden, 1992) have been shown to be useful with cancer patients. However, they must be used with a caveat when dealing with women. McGrath (1992) has found in her work with women and depression that cognitive methods, emphasizing the intellectual rather than the affective, tended to put women in the position of being told by an authority that they were not thinking correctly. These techniques have been found to be more effective with men, and overall, most cognitive practitioners tend to be male. At times, therefore, these interventions may be more suitable for the spouse of the patient.

With this caution in mind, we offer these techniques, some of which have valuable components. We remind practitioners that they must be used with sensitivity, especially with women who are already dealing with an authoritarian medical system. Typically these interventions are most effective following the initial crisis reaction, after the emotional upheaval has abated. Interventions can be done individually or in groups.

■ *COGNITIVE BEHAVIORAL STRATEGIES* – Golden's (Golden, Gersh, & Robbins, 1992) goal is to keep the cancer patient's life as normal as possible. He offers patients several cognitive techniques to combat the thinking patterns of depression—such as self-condemnation, hopelessness, and self-pity. Cognitive therapists distinguish between feelings of sadness and the experience of depression.

Whereas sadness is appropriate to the situation and motivates patients (e.g., to enjoy life as much as possible), depression is maladaptive and immobilizing. Cognitive therapists believe that depression is the result of faulty thinking, and their interventions are attempts to modify that system through self-monitoring and retraining.

Patients are taught to identify and rate their maladaptive thoughts. Practice sessions using evocative imagery (reexperiencing the actual thoughts and feelings) and therapeutic interventions attempt to replace the self-defeating patterns of thinking with more constructive, rational thought.

As part of this approach, the therapist may explore, in depth, a woman's beliefs about her own thoughts. Many women believe that thinking bad thoughts (pessimistic, fearful, anxious, or sad thoughts) will make them relapse or destroy the effectiveness of the treatment. Some breast cancer patients may also believe that their thoughts cause them to become ill, e.g., if they were angry, anxious, or unhappy prior to diagnosis.

Patients may need help in understanding the healthy free flow of thoughts and feelings which occur randomly and continuously in human beings, so that they feel more relaxed when frightening visual images cross their minds. It is useful to keep reminding patients that the goal is to reduce blocking, not to reduce bad thoughts. It may even be helpful at times to focus at length on "bad" thoughts, to discuss fears of becoming sicker, suffering, and dying. The therapist can help the patient notice how once the mind is satiated, "bad" thoughts are less frightening, and less prevalent. The mind begins to wander to happier, more optimistic ideas.

☞ *Examples of cognitive interventions:*

As if — *This technique can be effective for dealing with depression. The patient is instructed to act "as if" they felt different than they do. The idea is that if you behave in one way, the emotions will follow. A patient who is feeling worthless and hopeless is asked to behave as if she felt worthwhile. The worthwhile behaviors will then lead her to feel better about herself.*

Redefine goals — *Breaking up the "giveitupitis" by having the patient set attainable goals that they can master. For example, a patient may feel devastated that a planned European trip cannot take place. The therapist might help the patient redefine the goal ie. plan for a mini vacation that is attainable.*

Fight catastrophizations — *Help the patient replace a catastrophic response with a more rational one. For example, a patient may feel that the chemotherapy is not working, "The doctors have lied to me" (Catastrophic). The therapist might help the patient see that a more appropriate response could be "Some people require more treatment than others" or, "Doctors do not always know the outcome of treatments" (Rational).*

Focus on the quality of life — *Help the patient make every minute count. Set achievable goals. "Instead of waiting to die, let's set goals and see what we can accomplish."*

A note of caution — *One of the problems facing the therapist is how to "raise hope without instilling false hope...On the one hand, it is important to encourage positive thinking, although one also does not want to build false expectations...The therapist can make a distinction between using self-control procedures for coping with cancer and using them to cure cancer...It is important to help patients realize that it is a theory and not an established fact that cancer is either caused by depression or that cancer can be cured by psychological methods."*

(Golden et al., 1992, p. 25)

Facilitating a Breast Cancer Support Group

As noted in the chapter on support groups/group therapy, Frank (1992), has designed a structured group approach which she uses in one three-hour session with 16 participants. The group design presented here can easily be adapted for longer-term groups.

■ *OBJECTIVES OF THE GROUP* – Frank's group objectives are: 1) to open communication among participants concerning their experiences with breast cancer and 2) to provide emotional support and foster enhanced coping skills.

> ☞ *Each group consists of women who have undergone various treatments for different stages of breast cancer including mastectomy, lumpectomy, radiation or chemotherapy alone, or multiple treatments.*
>
> *The room is set up with separate tables, a flipchart, magic markers and masking tape. Light refreshments are available in the back of the room. The intent is to give the impression of serious work without the intensity or perceived threat of a therapy group.*

■ *INTRODUCTION: BUILDING A SUPPORTIVE CLIMATE* – It is important to set the tone immediately for an honest and forthright discussion. The group begins with the leader's introduction and explanation of his/her role as a psychologist with a particular interest in medical psychotherapy. (Frank suggests that as a model for self-disclosing behavior, she briefly offers some information about her relationship to the topic e.g., the discovery of a benign lump several years ago).

The psychologist then clarifies the leadership role, which is to facilitate a discussion of feelings, to identify and clarify the emotional issues, to build support for each other, and to discuss coping skills.

> ☞ *From the start, the facilitator needs to give clear directions and assert her authority, such as breaking in if someone speaks too long.*

■ *WHY AM I HERE? GROUP GO AROUND* – Each member of the group is asked to think about her answer to the question "Why am I here?" and to say a few words of self-introduction. The facilitator suggests that any comment will do but requests that each response be limited to one or two sentences. The facilitator signals for each person to begin, makes certain that no one person monopolizes the discussion, sets a supportive tone and offers a sense of leadership and safety.

☞ *None of the responses are challenged but are used to set parameters. For example, if a participant says she just came to hear what others have to say, the facilitator can suggest that everyone participate at their own level of comfort, but all are regarded as participants rather than observers.*

Throughout this group activity, the facilitator models the desired behavior of acceptance and respect for each person's contribution. Members usually introduce themselves by name, some mention careers, families or what kind of cancer they have had.

■ *EXPECTATIONS AND RESERVATIONS: DYADS* – Each group member is now asked to choose a partner, someone she did not know before she entered the room. These dyads are asked to discuss their expectations and reservations for the group session. They are told that in a few minutes, they will be asked to share these expectations and reservations, based on this discussion. Paper and pencil may be offered to help dyads focus.

☞ *This activity encourages the group to form alliances and begins the process of building group support for the larger discussion which follows.*

After the allotted time, participants are asked to verbalize the expectations and reservations discussed in the larger group. The facilitator records these responses on the flip chart.

☞ *Typical expectations are to discuss issues that people are afraid to talk about, to identify embarrassing feelings, to explore attitudes about fear, anger, and dying, and to hear how others handle intimacy.*

Typical reservations include: Will we trust each other? Do we want to risk exposure to others? Will we talk about just factual information? Who is the person who is the facilitator? (If the latter issue is not raised, Dr. Frank introduces it, as trust is vital in the initial stages of all groups. She feels it is particularly important in a group with a recent trauma experience. Typically, some members of the group may wonder whether anyone who has not had the experience of breast cancer can be helpful.)

Further group rules are then set, such as being able to ask each other any questions, but respecting the other's right not to answer. The facilitator suggests that the group be used as a laboratory to try out new behaviors and take some risks.

Without eliciting verbal responses, participants are asked to think about how open they felt during the initial discussion and to identify the thoughts that were not said out loud.

■ *WHAT HINDERS ME? AN EXERCISE FOR QUARTETS* – The dyads are asked to join together with another set of partners and to introduce each other. Four groups of four are thus formed to discuss the question, "What hinders me from dealing better emotionally with my breast cancer?" Each group, sitting around a table, is given a sheet from the flipchart and a magic marker. Participants are told they will be given 10-15 minutes to create a written list of responses and to decide who will report back to the larger group.

> ☞ *Typical responses include: body image, self expectation of being a superwoman, the "why me?" syndrome, recurring pain, arm swelling, poor self-concept, fear of rejection, stress, anxiety, other people's reactions, dealing with family, thinking that life will never be as good, anger, self pity, generalizations about "the cancer personality."*

Time is given for large group discussion after each subgroup has reported. If any typical responses are omitted, the leader may introduce them and ask for group comment. For example, participants often express feelings that medical professionals seem to stereotype the "cancer personality," and this makes them feel either blamed for their cancer or looked down upon.

At the end of the general discussion, the facilitator may ask these process questions:
1. Does your belief system hinder or help you to cope with breast cancer?
2. Can you identify dilemmas that have come up for you? (e.g.,desiring intimacy vs. needing privacy?)
3. What are the self-esteem issues which have arisen for you?
4. What are the emotional stages you have experienced?

To clarify this last question, the group is shown a list of commonly accepted stages of grief (from the work of Elizabeth Kubler- Ross, 1978) and told that any major loss in life might be applied to these stages. The stages are identified on the flipchart as denial, bargaining, anger, depression, and acceptance. In the larger group, members engage in an informal discussion abut these stages and suggest modifications in light of their own personal experience and self-observations.

> ☞ *Groups tend to modify the stages of grief as follows: panic, fear, self pity, fear, bargaining, anger, fear, depression, fear, acceptance, fear, trans- formation, and fear. The acknowledgment of fear and its intensity is essential for the success of the group.*

■ *WHAT HELPS ME DEAL MORE EFFECTIVELY WITH EMOTION? AN- OTHER QUARTET EXERCISE* – The groups of four continue (old or newly formed). Each group is asked to list responses to the question "What helps me deal better emotionally?" Another way to phrase this question is "What helps me to cope with breast cancer?"

Participants are asked to think about their coping skills and to categorize them. Is a coping technique physical, mental, emotional, social, or spiritual (e.g., a category that includes intuitive abilities)? What patterns tend to emerge?

■ *HOW MIGHT OTHERS HELP? QUARTETS* – According to Frank, this part of the design, while optional, has proven very valuable, and she suggests its inclusion. Once again, quartets are formed. Participants are asked, "How might others help?"

☞ *Answers are often specific and have included:*
- *Do specific chores such as chauffeuring, childcare, accompaniment to the physician.*
- *Ask probing questions.*
- *Accept my decisions about treatment.*
- *Continue to do activities that are enjoyable to both individuals.*
- *Set aside time to deal with the patient and her problems.*
- *Help the patient's children participate in the fighting process against the cancer.*
- *Keep your own stress under control and don't neglect yourself.*
- *Share your feelings and let me share mine.*

■ *ONE SMALL CHANGE: DYADS AND THE GROUP* – Original partners are asked to pair once again and to discuss the question, "What is one small behavioral change I want to make this week as a result of tonight's group?" Each woman is asked to share this answer with her partner.

In the large group now, each person takes a turn at revealing her newly developed goal. Because the changes stated are often too grandiose to be realistic, it is the job of the facilitator to suggest the change be minimized, when necessary, and specifically defined. In this way, each woman will have the possibility of reaching her goal.

☞ *For example, one woman may say she is making a commitment to exercise more. The facilitator may ask her to choose and agree to only one day in the coming week (although she is free to do more) and to define the exercise in a specific manner, e.g., walk at least 1/2 mile.*

The goal is that a very limited behavioral shift is an important step in the overall change process. It is suggested that each participant call her partner when her limited goal is attained.

Frank has found that this seven-stage design has been effective for opening discussion and facilitating the formation of supportive relationships. She encourages others to replicate this design in a three to four hour session or to spread the work out over three to four weeks.

Chapter 13
RESEARCH ON THE EFFECTIVENESS OF PSYCHOLOGICAL INTERVENTIONS

This section reviews the most significant research on the psychological treatment of breast cancer. In general, psychological interventions have been powerful adjuncts to medical treatments. Recent research on the psychological treatment of breast cancer has attempted to manipulate psychological factors during treatment in order to identify those interventions which lead to a positive outcome, e.g. increased survival time.

Psychological Interventions

■ *GROUP THERAPY* – Perhaps the most significant of the recent research studies is that of Spiegel, Bloom, Kraemer, & Gottheil (1989). Spiegel's et.al. metastatic breast cancer patients participated in weekly group psychotherapy with hypnosis for pain and routine oncological care. Eight months after the intervention, the two groups began to diverge in outcome, with the treatment group surviving twice as long as the control group. Several of the treatment subjects were still alive at the end of the ten-year study.

> ☞ *Spiegel's et. al. groups met weekly in outpatient settings for 90 minutes and were made up of 7-10 women. Although his research study lasted only one year, the groups elected to continue on after this time. Each group had two leaders, a psychiatrist or a social worker and a counselor who had breast cancer in remission. Leaders received prior training, and met regularly after each group meeting. Increased survival time was the most important outcome. Additional benefits of group participation were a reduction in depression (hypothesized to improve health care), an increase in healthy routines, and an improvement in relationships with friends and family. Spiegel's groups appeared to enhance immune functions, slow the progression of the disease and provide a powerful source of social support for the members.*
>
> *Other research supports these conclusions. Weisman & Worden (1975) found beneficial effects (i.e. living significantly longer) in patients who maintained cooperative and mutually responsive relationships.*

■ *INDIVIDUAL PSYCHOTHERAPY* – Grossarth-Maticek and Eysenck (1989) provided individual psychotherapy to women with metastasized breast cancer and found that survival time improved by 50% across all types of psychotherapy.

■ *DEVELOPING RELATIONSHIP SKILLS* – The existence of supportive relationships is a key factor in the psychological treatment of breast cancer. For example,
survival from breast cancer was predictable after four years, in part, from the number
of supportive friends and other persons in the patient's life (Waxler-Morrison, Hislop,
Mears, & Kan, 1991). "There is little evidence in our findings that relationships within
the woman's family and with her relatives are important for survival. Instead, the social
contexts that appear to be significant are outside the woman's home" (p.180). The data
indicate that the concrete help given by friends was an important predictor of outcome,
even though family help may be present and substantial. The "colleague network" which
women describe as occurring through employment networks was particularly important.

Eysenck and Grossarth-Maticek (1991) provided a behavioral group treatment to
teach interpersonal skills to cancer-prone patients. When group members were surveyed
after seven years, 7.5% of the treated, cancer-prone group and 47.4% of the untreated
control group had died, supporting the importance of interpersonal relationships.

■ *SUPPORT GROUPS* – Positive social relationships optimize the likelihood of a good
prognosis with breast cancer, and so any source of social relating is often encouraged.
However, the research data reviewed in this manual apply only to professionally led
psychotherapy groups. These professional groups, unlike "self-help or lay support
groups", are well-constructed, form part of a larger treatment approach, and are led by
experienced, trained leaders. Programs offered by the American Cancer Society, such as
Reach to Recovery, and others which counsel women, provide information, arrange
contacts with other patients, offer hope, help or companionship, can presumably be of
great utility to many women, although they are not true psychotherapy groups.

■ *HYPNOSIS* – Hypnosis is an excellent tool in helping the breast cancer patient to weather the experience of illness and treatment. Hypnosis can rapidly bypass the repressive defenses and offer relief from symptoms. The technique of analogue marking, for example, identifies certain words or phrases for the patient nonverbally, by voice tone or pacing, in order to directly access the subconscious and elicit a cooperative response from the constructive part of the psyche.

> ☞ *Hypnosis produces an altered state of consciousness, and helps the cancer patient deal with unpleasant somatic and emotional responses, including pain, nausea, vomiting and anxiety. The teaching of self-hypnosis to help the patient master pain outside the treatment setting may use many forms of instruction. Spiegel (1985) for example, teaches breast cancer patients not to fight the pain, but to "filter the hurt out of the pain" and imagine such sensations as icy cold numbness, or warm tingling. Patients can be induced to develop anesthesia in various body parts, or to produce a change in body temperature in one or another location, as for example, when patients use the visual image of a warm bath to one or another body part.*
>
> *The shifting of attention to nonpainful body parts (Spiegel, 1985) or a pairing of pain relief instructions with a classically conditioned stimulus such as a telephone call (Clawson & Swade, 1975) may summon up untapped resources in the patient to deal more productively with pain. These types of inductions seem to be particularly effective when combined with group psychotherapy. A sensitive ear to the patient is important in using these techniques, as she may not want to disappoint the therapist with continuing symptoms.*
>
> *Hypnotic techniques appear to offer help to cancer patients in the reduction of pain, although their overall success depends on the hypnotizability of the patients. In general, they appear to reduce pain in about half of cancer patients (Cangello, 1961; Lea, Ware, & Monroe, 1960).*
>
> *The experience of nausea and vomiting, so common with chemotherapy, may be further complicated by the appearance of anticipatory nausea and vomiting occuring in about 25% of cancer patients. This experience is one in which the patient develops side effects as treatment approaches, as well as while treatment is underway. These responses appear to develop as a result of stimulus generalization, and may occur more often in later chemotherapy cycles. Hypnosis can be therapeutic, when patients are taught to focus attention, achieve deep muscle relaxation and visualize relaxing scenes, with daily practice using taped instructions (Redd, Andersen, & Minagawa, 1982). Spiegel (1985) suggests to his patients that they deliver their body but not their mind for treatment, concentrating during a trance on pleasant experiences while medical treatment is given so as to separate psychological reactions from somatic distress.*
>
> *A full range of hypnotic inductions and instructions are available elsewhere (Grindler, 1981) but require training in both hypnotherapy and psychotherapy for safe usage. The physiological consequences of using hypnotic techniques, as for example in changing blood flow (Clawson, 1975) and other measures make it imperative that the therapist have good training in the use of these tools with medical/surgical patients. It is also valuable to have a clear understanding of the patient's psychological status before utilizing hypnotic techniques in order not to compromise emotional stability.*

■ *PROGRESSIVE RELAXATION* – Progressive relaxation and meditation, two overlapping techniques, both of which are sometimes regarded as forms of self-hypnosis, can be useful in the control of pain, nausea, and anxiety. The former involves a sequence of deep muscle relaxation, followed by guided imagery (Benson, 1975). Muscle relaxation may involve the imagining of temperature, weight, or tension changes as well.

> ☞ *Research results generally support the effectiveness of these treatments in reducing nausea and vomiting, as well as anxiety, pulse rate and blood pressure (Lyles, Burish, Krozely, & Oldham, 1982). Their effectiveness seems to depend upon the presence of the therapist. The research suggests that progressive relaxation is contraindicated with patients who have a serious psychological disorder, those with counter-phobic reactions, some personality disorders, and patients with certain types of diffuse nervous pain. Although the use of tapes with progressive relaxation training is routine, it may be problematic with breast cancer patients, because it may increase their sense of emotional isolation and responsibility for their difficulties.*

■ *SYSTEMATIC DESENSITIZATION* – This counterconditioning technique is generally used as part of a behavior regimen. It has traditionally been used to treat phobias and anxiety disorders. The therapist constructs with the patient a hierarchy of progressively more aversive images. The hierarchy might begin, for example, with an imagined phone call to arrange the next chemotherapy treatment, moving to the most aversive image, perhaps that of painful or emetic reactions to treatment. In a state of deep muscle relaxation, the patient moves along the hierarchy step by step, practicing the retention of the relaxed state in the face of increasingly provocative stimuli.

Research indicates that systematic desensitization is more effective than Rogerian counseling in reducing the frequency, severity, and duration of anticipatory nausea and vomiting in cancer patients (Morrow, 1982). When patients are treated with this technique early in the chemotherapy series, it appears to reduce conditioned side effects (Dobkin, Zeichner, & Dickson-Parnell, 1985).

Some of the difficulty with these techniques to control post-chemotherapy reactions, concerns the powerful effect of the chemical substances. There is the risk of aversive reaction becoming conditioned to secondary stimuli, so that the therapist begins to elicit nausea/vomiting.

■ *BIOFEEDBACK* – Biofeedback consists of a technique that directly monitors the body's physiological arousal, and generally involves some mechanical registering of the patient's bodily sensations. This may be used in conjunction with other methods, most often with visual imagery. When biofeedback is used to increase relaxation during the administration of chemotherapy, patients reported that anxiety and nausea were both reduced (Burish, Shartner, & Lyles, 1981). Like other techniques of this kind, biofeedback can serve to enhance the patient's sense of control over her body.

■ **PHYSIOLOGICAL EVIDENCE OF PSYCHOLOGICAL TREATMENTS** – Two theories have been proposed to account for the appearance, spread and reduction of malignant cells. The first, a theory of immunosurveillance, suggests that randomly appearing cancer cells are routinely destroyed by T lymphocytes, including natural killer cells. The second is an explanation based on endocrinological influences in combination with various protective responses, themselves greatly affected by psychological states. The latter approach holds particular relevance for breast cancer, since estrogen, androgen, and prolactin levels have a clear influence on the course of the disease.

Alternative explanations of immune functions focus on the effect of emotional reactions on the mobilization of free fatty acids, or on local rather than system-wide factors, similar to the localized effects of hypnosis on wart tissue.

■ **NATURAL KILLER CELLS** – Levy, Herberman, Maluish, Schlien, & Lippman (1985), have found natural killer cell activity level to be related to long-term survival in breast cancer patients. Natural killer cell activity level was itself predictable from levels of social support (Levy, Herberman, Shiteside, Sanzo, Lee, & Kirkwood, 1990). In Stage I and Stage II breast cancer patients, the perception of high-quality support from a spouse, or intimate other, or emotional support from medical caregivers, were powerful predictors of natural killer cell activity level. This finding suggests that the connection between social support and health status may be mediated by certain types of T cells.

Levy and Wise (1988) examined the effects of depressive pessimism and helplessness on breast cancer patients. Helplessness was defined as the attribution of personal negative experiences to internal, stable, and global causes, as shown in the statement, "This kind of thing always happens to me". They found that helplessness indices were associated with earlier disease recurrence.

■ **EFFECTS OF LIFE CHANGE ON IMMUNE FUNCTION** – The immune response to psychological influences has led some researchers (Blalock, Harbour-McMenamin, & Smith, 1985) to propose that the immune system be considered a sensory organ. The immune system apparently registers psychological events in a measurable way, so that when a spouse dies (Bartrop, Luckhurst, Kiloh, & Penny, 1977), or decides to separate from the marriage (Kiecolt-Glaser, Fisher, Ogrocki, Stout, Speicher, & Glaser, 1987), the remaining partner shows poorer function on immunological assays, with short separation and close attachment inversely related to the immune measures. Chronic stressors, such as the responsibility for caring for an ill, older relative predict poorer immune function (Kiecolt-Glaser et al, 1987) as do cataclysmic community events (McKinnon, Weisse, Reynolds, Bowles, & Baum, 1989).

Research has shown a rise in immune measures when psychotherapeutic treatment is offered to cancer patients. Fawzi (1990) found substantial positive changes in immune function after a six-week group mental health intervention. Similarly, Eysenck and Grossarth-Maticek's (1991) individual psychotherapy treatment produced increases in lymphocyte function for metastatic breast cancer patients.

Other findings indicate that changes in psychological setting seem to improve immune function. When older adults are given relaxation training, there is a rise in natural killer cell activity (Kiecolt-Glaser, et al., 1987), and when college students are asked to regularly write about traumatic, secret memories, they show improved immune function, and make fewer visits to the college infirmary (Pennebaker, 1988).

Chapter 14
RESOURCES

The following list covers a variety of resources available to psychologists working with breast cancer patients and their families.

Resources for Psychologists

■ **The National Cancer Institute**
1-800-4-CANCER

This diverse organization is funded by the U.S. Department of Health and Human Services, and offers the following:

• *A series of pamphlets entitled the Breast Cancer Patient Education Series.*
Office of Cancer Communications
National Cancer Institute
Building 31, Room 10A24
Bethesda, Maryland 20892

• *A paperback handbook called The Breast Cancer Digest: A Guide to Medical Care, Emotional Support, Educational Programs, and Resources.*
U.S. Department of Health & Human Services
Public Health Service
National Institutes of Health
NCI
Bethesda, Maryland 20205

• *An extensive listing of materials and publications, including Cancergram, a review of current research literature.*
Office of Cancer Communications
Building 31, Room 10A-16
Bethesda, Maryland 20892
301/496-5583 (professionals only)

The information listed below may be obtained by calling 1-800-4- CANCER

• *Cancer Information Service: Trained specialists are available to answer questions in English and Spanish.*

• *Clinical Community Oncology Program (CCOP). This is a list of community programs in 31 states that participate in NCI research on cancer treatments and accept patients for experiment participation.*

• *PDQ (Physician's Data Query). This is a computerized information service which gives current information on breast cancer publications, physicians, and treatment centers.*

■ **National Alliance of Breast Cancer Organizations (NABCO)**
1180 Avenue of the Americas,
Second Floor
New York, NY 10036

This organization functions in two ways:

• *Information clearinghouse: NABCO provides individuals and organizations with current information about breast cancer detection and treatment. It publishes* the extensive Breast Cancer Resource List, which is an exhaustive survey of books, pamphlets, organizations, videos, and so forth.

• *Lobby and Advocacy: NABCO acts to influence public and private health policy on breast cancer.*

■ **National Surgical Breast Adjuvant and Bowel Project (NSABP)**
3550 Terrace Street, Room 914
Pittsburgh, PA 15261
412/648-9720
• *NSABP maintains a listing of physicians participating in clinical trials and* will provide information by area.

■ **The Komen Alliance**
1-800-IMAWARE
214-980-8841
• *This is a memorial program for the research, education and treatment of breast cancer. Information and resources available on request.*

■ **AMC Cancer Research Center's Cancer Information Line**
1-800-525-3777
• *Counselors with training will provide information and support regarding cancer.*

Resources for Patients

■ **American Cancer Society**
1-800-ACS-2345
Tower Place
3340 Peachtree Road NE
Atlanta, GA 30026
• *This is a volunteer organization which has chapters in most communities, and offers patients and families various programs and supports, such as transportation, equipment loan and rental, support groups and informational help.*

■ **Cancer Information Service**
1-800-4-CANCER
• *The cancer information service, available in English and Spanish, provides up-to-date information on cancer to patients and their families. Information is offered on the latest cancer treatments, clinical trials, tips on early detection and risk reduction, and community services for patients and families. Free booklets on cancer can be ordered.*

■ **Reach To Recovery**
(under the American Cancer Society)
1-800-ACS-2345
• *This service is offered locally by chapters and has volunteers who are recovered breast cancer patients who are trained to offer help and support. Hospital visits (must be arranged through the physician) and home visits are offered. Also monthly meetings.*

■ **I Can Cope**
(under the American Cancer Society)
1-800-ACS-2345
• *This is a program aimed at the educational support of patients and their families, and provides help in understanding treatment, therapy, side effects, etc.*

■ **Cancer Care, Inc.**
212-221-3300
1180 Avenue of the Americas
New York, NY 10036

• *Cancer Care is a non-profit, non-sectarian agency which offers professional individual, family, and group counseling at no cost to cancer patients, their families and friends. Direct services is available in New York, New Jersey and Connecticut. Callers from other parts of the country will be advised of local services in their community. A number of helpful pamphlets are available from Cancer Care, Inc.*

■ **Encore (Encouragement, Normalcy, Counseling, Opportunity, Reaching Out Energies Revived)**
YWCA National Headquarters
726 Broadway
New York, NY 10003
212-614-2827
• *Organized by the YWCA, Encore offers discussion groups for post-operative breast cancer patients, and information. Contact the national association for local services.*

■ **Y-ME National Organization for Breast Cancer Information and Support**
18220 Harwood Avenue
Homewood, IL 60430
800-221-2141 or 708-799-8228
• *This is a national, non-profit organization that offers help and support to callers by trained volunteers, many of whom have had breast cancer. In the Chicago area, and some other cities, there are monthly support meetings.*

■ **Make Today Count**
P.O. Box 22
Osage Beach, MO 65065
314-348-1619
• *Aimed at the broad population of patients with life-threatening illnesses, this organization uses a buddy system for peer support, and concentrates on improving the quality of life.*

■ **The National Coalition of Cancer Survivorship**
1010 Wayne Aenue, Fifth Floor
Silver Spring, MD 20910
301-650-8868
• *This is a network of independent organizations and individuals which focuses on survivor issues and helps patients and their families locate services. It is an information bank, as well as a peer support and advocacy organization.*

■ **The Susan G. Komen Breast Cancer Foundation**
6820 LBJ Freeway, Suite 130
Dallas, TX 75240
1-800-IMAWARE
• *This organization offers information on screening, treatment and support, and offers help in locating mammography facilities.*

■ **RENU Breast Reconstruction Counseling**
215-456-7383
• *For women considering reconstruction, this program offers trained counselors who are volunteers who have had reconstruction. It is part of the Einstein Medical Center in Philadelphia.*

■ **Cancer Research Council**
301-654-7933
4853 Cordell Avenue, Suite 11
Bethesda, Maryland 20814
• *This organization focuses on new medical treatment concepts currently in the experimental stage, and will send information.*

■ **National Consumer Insurance Helpline**
1-800-942-4242

■ **The Wellness Community**
1-800-PRO-HOPE
1235 Fifth Street
Santa Monica, CA 90401
• *This is a center for a series of support and education programs that focus more on creating healthy life than on defeating disease.*

■ **Corporate Angel Network**
914-328-1313
Westchester County Airport, Bldg. 1
White Plains, NY 10604
• *An unusual organization which offers help to patients traveling to NCI-approved treatment facilities by providing transportation to patients on corporate aircraft on routine flights where available.*

Mass Market Books on Breast Cancer

Brinker, Nancy. **The Race is Run One Step at a Time: Everywoman's Guide to Taking Charge of Breast Cancer.** Simon and Schuster, 1990.

The author is the sister of Susan Komen, a breast cancer patient, in whose memory the Komen Foundation was created. The book is a good but brief guide for the patients to the major issues an decisions of the breast cancer patient.

Fabian, Carol & Warren, Andrea. **Recovering from Breast Cancer: A Doctor's Guide for Women and Their Families.** New York: Harper Paperbacks, 1992.

This is part of Harper's Recovering From Diseases Series and gives basic information about breast cancer treatment. It has two sections on recovery, physical and emotional, and offers more psychological coverage than most guidebooks on this topic.

Hirshaut, Y. & Pressman, P.I. **Breast Cancer: The Complete Guide**. New York: Bantam Books, 1992.

An excellent, readable book on the treatment of breast cancer written by a breast surgeon and an oncologist. Particularly helpful is the step-by-step review of the treatment process. Also, there is a rare explanation of the drugs used for chemotherapy, their uses and various side effects.

Kahane, Deborah. **No Less A Woman**. New York: Prentice Hall Press, 1990.

Ten women talk about their breast cancer, how it affected their lives and their feelings. An excellent work for illustrating the range of reactions.

Kaye, Ronnie. **Spinning Straw Into Gold: Your Emotional Recovery From Breast Cancer**. New York: Simon & Schuster, 1991.

Good exploration of the psychological issues and effects surrounding breast cancer treatment and recovery, done with examples from the author's clinical and personal experience.

LeShan, Lawrence. **Cancer As a Turning Point: A Handbook for People With Cancer, Their Families, and Health Professionals**. New York: E.P. Dutton, 1989.

Part of the older work in cancer that tries to get patients to make decisions about life issues that become more pressing with a cancer diagnosis. LeShan is a pioneer in this area, and his work is well worth reading.

Love, Susan. **Dr. Susan Love's Breast Book**. New York: Addison-Wesley, 1990.

The author is a breast surgeon who clearly and carefully reviews the medical issues involved with breast cancer diagnosis and treatment. This book is well written, but it is not a "quick read." Patients can be directed to specific sections, e.g. "Diagnosis and Types of Cancer" or "Treatment Options".

Morra, M. & Potts, E. **Choices: Realistic Alternatives in Cancer Treatment**. New York: Avon Books, 1987.

Many different kinds of cancers are addressed in this book (e.g. skin cancer, lung cancer etc), but the chapters on radiation, chemotherapy and breast cancer are particularly well written and appropriate for breast cancer patients. The writing style is an easy question and answer format. There are also a number of tables in the breast cancer chapter which lead the patient through medical processes in a step-by-step progression with appropriate explanations.

Nessim, Susan & Ellis, Judith. **Cancervive: The Challenge of Life After Cancer**. New York: Houghton Mifflin, 1991.

Covers all cancers, but focuses on the psychological issues after treatment. A good piece that offers many specific stories. The basis for Cancervive, the non-profit organization offering support to long term cancer survivors.

Seligman, Martin. **Learned Optimism**. New York: Simon & Schuster, 1990.

Probably the best work available in mass market on how to change cognitive patterns. Very useful for cancer patients interested in dealing with psychological issues.

Siegel, B.S. **Love, Medicine and Miracles**. New York: Harper and Row, 1986.

This book, at one time on the best seller list, is included because many patients have already read it or have heard of it. The subject of the book is the interrelationship between the mind and the body, and the patient's ability to take charge of his/her health. Unfortunately, the material is presented in a manner that can foster guilt and self blame. Patients can easily come away with the message that their illness is "all their fault". This is, all too often, the unfortunate outcome of reading this book.

Chapter 15
SELECTED MEDICAL GLOSSARY

(adapted from Hermann, Wojtkowiak, Houts, & Kahn, 1991; Love, 1991)

ADJUVANT TREATMENT — treatments that are added to increase the effectiveness of the primary treatment. This usually refers to radiation or chemotherapy after surgery, used to increase the likelihood of a cure.

ALOPECIA — hair loss; a common side effect of chemotherapy, usually temporary.

AUTOLOGOUS BONE MARROW TRANSPLANT (ABMT) — a still- experimental technique of administering massive doses of chemotherapy in a hospital setting which intensively destroys cancer cells as well as depressing the person's immune system. The patient's bone marrow, which manufactures blood cells, is harvested for possible future use.

AXILLARY LYMPH NODE DISSECTION — surgical removal of lymph nodes found in the armpit region.

BENIGN TUMOR — an abnormal growth that is not cancerous and does not spread to other areas of the body.

BIOPSY — the surgical removal of a small piece of tissue for examination of cancer cells. Used in the diagnosis of cancer.

CARCINOMA IN SITU — an early stage of highly curable cancer which is confined to the tissue of origin.

CEA (CARCINOEMBRYONIC ANTIGEN) — a nonspecific (not specific to cancer) blood test used to follow women with metastatic breast cancer to help determine if the treatment is effective. CEA can be followed over time and will often be elevated if metastasis develop.

CHEMOTHERAPY — treatment of cancer by use of drugs. Some typical drugs are adriamycin, cyclophosphamide, methotrexate, and 5-fluorouracil.

CLINICAL TRIAL — experimental studies using new methods of treatment for cancer. Patients need to qualify to be subjects in a clinical trial. Patients have the right to refuse to be part of such a study.

CYST — an abnormal structure that contains liquid or semi-solid material. A cyst may be benign or malignant. Lumps in the breast are often found to be harmless cysts.

CYTOXIC — Causing the death of cells. The term usually refers to drugs used in chemotherapy.

EDEMA — Swelling caused by a collection of fluid in the soft tissues.

FROZEN SECTION — Procedure often done during surgery to diagnose cancer. Tissue is removed by biopsy, then it is frozen, cut, stained and examined under a microscope.

HIGH RISK — The chances of developing cancer are greater than normally seen in the general population, e.g., women whose mothers have had breast cancer are at higher risk of developing it themselves.

IMMUNOTHERAPY — a treatment that stimulates the body's own defense mechanisms in combating cancer.

LOCALIZED CANCER — A cancer that is still confined to its site of origin.

LYMPH NODES — glands that act as the filters of impurities throughout the body. Lymph nodes can be a location of cancer spread.

MALIGNANT TUMOR — cancer cells that may invade surrounding tissues or spread throughout the body.

MAMMOGRAPHY — a screening and diagnostic procedure that uses low-dose X-rays to find tumors in the breast. Mammography reveals tumors that are too small to be felt by touch (palpated).

METASTASIS — the spread of cancer cells to distant areas of the body by way of the lymph system or bloodstream.

MICROMETASTASIS — microscopic and as yet undetectable (but presumed) spread of tumor cells to other organs.

ONCOLOGIST — physicians who specialize in the treatment of cancer. The medical team will often consist of the oncologist who manages the overall treatment and administers chemotherapy, a breast surgeon, and a radiation therapist.

PALLIATIVE TREATMENT — therapy that is used to relieve symptoms (e.g., pain), but does not alter the course of the disease. Its primary purpose is to improve the quality of life.

PRECANCEROUS — abnormal cellular changes that are potentially capable of becoming cancer. These lesions are amenable to treatment and cure. Also called premalignant.

RADIOTHERAPY — the treatment of cancer with high-energy radiation. Radiation therapy may be used to reduce the size of a cancer before surgery, or to destroy remaining cancer cells after surgery. Radiotherapy can be helpful in shrinking recurrent cancers to relieve symptoms.

RECURRENCE (LOCAL) — the reappearance of cancer at its original site after a period of remission.

REMISSION — complete or partial disappearance of the signs and symptoms of disease in response to treatment. The period during which a disease is under control. A remission is not necessarily a cure.

SYSTEMIC TREATMENT — treatment involving the whole body, usually using drugs.

TAMOXIFEN — a type of hormonal or sytemic therapy that is particularly effective with post-menopausal women. It is given in pill form and has minimal side effects.

TITRATION — systems of balancing. In chemotherapy titration means using the largest amount of a drug possible while keeping the side effects from becoming intolerable.

TNM SYSTEM — a staging system that groups tumors according to the extent of the disease. TNM stands for tumor, nodes and metastasis. The criteria are the size of the tumor, the presence of cancer cells in the lymph nodes, and the spread of the cancer to other sites. The staging system will help determine the course of treatment.

TRAM-flap (TRANSVERSE RECTUS ABDOMINUS MYOCUTANEOUS) — a type of breast reconstruction using the patient's abdominal tissue.

TUMOR — an abnormal tissue swelling or mass; may be either benign or malignant.

ULTRASOUND EXAMINATION — the use of high-frequency sound waves to locate a tumor deep inside the body.

SELECTED REFERENCES

Medical Treatment

Benson, H. (1985). *Beyond the relaxation response.* New York: Berkley Books.

Bovberg, D. (1990). Psychoneuroimmunology and cancer. In J.C. Holland and J.H. Rolland (Eds.), *Handbook of psychooncology* (pp. 727 - 734). New York: Oxford University Press.

Department of Labor, Health and Human Services, and Education and Related Agencies Appropriation Bill, 1992, *Report 102-104,* calendar No. 153, bill H.R. 2707., Washington, DC, July 11, 1991.

Grossarth-Maticek, R. & Eysenck, H.J. (1989). Length of survival and lympho-cyte percentage in women with mammary cancer as a function of psychotherapy. *Psychological Reports*, 1989, *65*, 315-321.

Hermann, J.F., Wojtkowiak, S.L., Houts, P.S., & Kahn, S. B. (1990) *Helping people cope.* Handout available through Cancer Care, New York, NY.

Hirshaut, Y. & Pressman, P.I. (1992). *Breast cancer: The complete guide.* New York: Bantam Books.

Holland, J.C. & Lesko, L.M. (1990). Chemotherapy, endocrine therapy, and immunotherapy. In J.C. Holland & J.H. Rowland (Eds.), *Handbook of psychooncology* (pp. 146-163). New York: Oxford University Press.

Lourde, A. (1980). *The cancer journals.* Spinsters/Aunt Lute, San Francisco.

Love, S. (1990). *Dr. Susan Love's breast book.* Addison-Wesley Publishing Company: Woburn, MA.

National Cancer Institute. (1990). *Questions and answers about breast lumps.* (NIH Pamphlet No. 90-2401). Washington, DC: U.S. Printing Office.

National Cancer Institute (1989). *Breast biopsy: What you need to know.* (NIH Publication No. 90-657). Washington, DC: U.S. Printing Office

Rolland, J.H. & Holland, J.C. (1990). Breast cancer. In J.C. Holland and J.H. Rolland (Eds.), *Handbook of psychooncology* (pp. 188-207). New York: Oxford University Press.

Siegel, B. S. (1986). *Love, medicine and miracles.* New York: Harper and Row.

Simonton, O., Mathews-Simonton, S., & Creighton, J. (1980). *Getting well again*. New York: Bantam Books.

Spiegel, D., & Bloom, J.R. (1983). Group therapy and hypnosis reduce metastic breast carcinoma pain. *Psychosomatic Medicine, 4*, 333-339.

Spiegel, D., Bloom, J.R., Kraemer, H.C., & Gottheil, E. (1989). Effect of psychosocial treatment on survival of patients with metastatic breast cancer. *The Lancet, #8668*, p. 888-891.

The Relationships Among Patient, Physician, and Psychologist

American Cancer Society. (1987). *Talking with your doctor*. (4638 PS Handout).

Broadhead, W.E. & Kaplan, B. (1991). Social support and cancer patients. *Cancer, 67* (suppl.).

Foley, K. (1985). Cancer Pain. In R.T. Johnson (Ed.) *Current therapy in neurologic disease*. Philadelphia: B.C. Decker.

National Coalition for Cancer Survivorship (1990). *Breast reconstruction after mastectomy*. (NIH Publication No. 91-2151) Washington, DC: U.S. Printing Office.

Portenoy, R.K. & Foley, K.M. (1990). Management of cancer pain. In J.C. Holland & J.H. Rowland (Eds.), *Handbook of psychooncology* (pp. 188-297). New York: Oxford University Press.

Rowland, J.H., & Holland, J.C. (1990). Breast cancer. In J.C. Holland & J.H. Roland (Eds.), *Handbook of psychooncology* (pp. 188-207). New York: Oxford University Press.

Spiegel, D. (1990). Facilitating emotional coping during treatment. *Cancer, 66*, 1422-1426.

Psychological Reactions To Diagnosis & Treatment

Bailar, J., & Smith, E. (1986). Progress against cancer? *New England Journal of Medicine 314*, 1226-1232.

Brownell, K. (1991). Personal responsibility and control over our bodies: When expectation exceeds reality. *Health Psychology, 10*, 303-310.

Fentiman, I., Cuzick, J., Millis, R., & Hayward, J. (1984). Which patients are cured of breast cancer? *British Medical Journal, 289,* 1108-1111.

Ganz, P.A., Polinsky, M.L., Schag, C.A.C., & Heinrich, R.L. (1989). Rehabilitation of patients with primary breast cancer: Assessing the impact of adjuvant therapy. In A.J. Senn (Ed.), *Adjuvant therapy of primary breast cancer.* New York: Springer Velag.

Gingrich, R., Burns, L., Wen, B., & Clamon, G. (1991). A phase I/II study of high-dose chemotherapy with marrow stem cell support in advanced breast cancer. *Proceedings of the Annual Meeting of the American Society of Clinical Onocology* 10:A142.

Holland, J.C. & Lesko, L.M. (1990). Chemotherapy, endocrine therapy, and immunotherapy (pp. 146-163). In J.C. Holland & J.H. Rowland (Eds.), *Handbook of psychooncology.* New York: Oxford University Press.

Hopwood, P., Howell, A., & Maguire, P. (1991). Psychiatric morbidity in patients with advanced breast cancer. *British Journal of Cancer, 2,* 349-52.

Lichtin, A., Weick, J., Andresen, S., Burwell, R., Sands, K., Murar, A., Bauer, L., Fishleder, A., Green, R., & Bolwell, B. (1991). Treatment of metastatic breast cancer with high-dose chemotherapy followed by autologous bone marrow transplantation (ABMT). *Proceedings of the Annual Meeting of the American Society of Clinical Oncology* 10:A90.

Lourde, A. (1980). *The cancer journals.* San Francisco: Spinsters/Aunt Lute.

Loveys, B. & Klaich, K. (1991). Breast cancer: demands of illness. *Oncology Nursing Forum, 18,* 75-80.

Memorial Sloan-Kettering-64th Street. (October 1992). Fact Sheet. Available from the public relations office, Memorial Sloan-Kettering Cancer Center. New York, NY.

Meyerwoitz, B. (1980). Psychosocial correlates to breast cancer and its treatments. *Psychological Bulletin , 87,* 108-131.

Meyerowitz, B.E., Watkins, I.K., & Sparks, F.C. (1983). Psychosocial implications of adjuvant chemotherapy, a two year followup. *Cancer, 52,* 1541-1545.

Rolland, J.H. & Holland, J.C. (1990). Breast cancer. In J.C. Holland, & J.H. Rolland (Eds.), *Handbook of psychooncology* (pp. 188-207). New York: Oxford University Press.

Spiegel, D. (1990). Facilitating emotional coping during treatment. *Cancer, 66* (6), (Suppl. Sept. 15), 1422-1426.

Skrabanek, P. (1985). False premises and false promises of breast cancer screening. *The Lancet, #8450*, p. 316-319.

Psychological Reactions— Posttreatment

Derogatis, L. R., Abeloff, M., & Melisaratos, N. (1979). Psychological coping mechanisms and survival in metastatic breast cancer. *Journal of the American Medical Association, 242,* 1504-1508.

Easterling, D.V. & Leventhal, H. (1989). Contribution of concrete cognition to emotion: Neutral symptoms as elicitors of worry about cancer. *Journal of Applied Psychology, 74,* 787-796.

Greer, S., Morris, T., & Pettingale, K.W. (1979). Psychological response to breast cancer: Effect on outcome. *Lancet, 13,* 785-787.

Kaplan, H.S. (1992). A neglected issue: The sexual side effects of current treatments for breast cancer. *Journal of Sex and Marital Therapy, 18,* 3-19.

Levy, S., Herberman, R., Lippman, M., & d'Angelo, T. (1987). Correlation of natural killer cell activity and predicted prognosis in patients with breast cancer. *Journal of Clinical Oncology, 5,* 348-353.

Levy, S., Herberman, R., Maluish A., Schlien, B., & Lippman, M. (1985). Prognostic risk assessment in primary breast cancer by behavioral and immunological parameters. *Health Psychology, 4,* 99-113.

Levy, S., Lee, J., Bagley, C., & Lippman, M. (1988) Survival hazards analysis in first recurrent breast cancer patients: Seven-year follow-up. *Psychosomatic Medicine, 50,* 520-528.

Levy, S., & Wise, B. (1988). Psychological risk factors and cancer progression. In C.L. Cooper (Ed.), *Stress and breast cancer* (pp. 77-96). John Wiley & Sons Ltd.

Mendelsohn, G.A. (1991). Psychosocial adaptation to illness by women with breast cancer and women with cancer at other sites. *Journal of Psychosocial Oncology, 8,* 1-25.

Meyerowitz, B.E., Watkins, I.K., & Sparks, F.C. (1983). Psychosocial implications of adjuvant chemotherapy: A two year follow-up. *Cancer, 52,* 1541-1545.

Nelson, D.V., Freidman, L.C., Baer, P.E., Lane, M., & Smith, F.E. (1989). Attitude to cancer: Psychometric properties of fighting spirit and denial. *Journal of Behavioral Medicine, 12,* 341-355.

Reynolds, P., & Kaplan, G. (1986, March). *Social connections and cancer: A prospective study of Alameda County residents.* Paper presented at the meeting of the Society of Behavioral Medicine, San Francisco, CA.

Rovner, S. (1987, March 17). Breast cancer: More cases, more treatments, more decisions (Health section). *The Washington Post,* pp. 12-17.

Spiegel, D. (1990). Can psychotherapy prolong cancer survival? *Psychosomatic Medicine, 31,* 361-366.

Watson, M. (1988). Breast cancer: Psychological factors influencing progression. In C.L. Cooper (Ed.), *Stress and breast cancer* (pp. 65-75). John Wiley & Sons Ltd.

Waxler-Morrison, N., Hislop, T.G., Mears, B., & Kan, L. (1991). Effects of social relationships on survival for women with breast cancer: A prospective study. *Social Science Medicine, 33,* 177-183.

Recurrence and Terminal Illness

Levy, S. (1985). *Behavior and cancer.* San Francisco: Jossey-Bass.

Linn, M.W., Linn, B.S. & Harris, R. (1982). Effects of counseling for late stage cancer patients. *Cancer, 49,* 1048-1055.

Lourde, A. (1980). *The cancer journals.* New York: Spinsters/Aunt Lute.

Speigel, D. & Yalom, I.D. (1978). A support group for dying patients. *International Journal of Group Psychotherapy, 28,* 233-245.

St. Francis Center. (1991). *Interventions for caregivers.* Washington, D.C. (Handout).

Wagener, J. & Taylor, S. (1986). What else could I have done? Patients' responses to failed treatment decisions. *Health Psychology, 5,* 481-496.

Weisman, A.D. & Worden, J.W. (1975). Psychosocial analysis of cancer deaths. *Omega, 6,* 61-75.

Patient - Psychologist Relationship

Cancer Care's Pain Resource Center. Pamphlet available from Cancer Care, Inc., New York, NY.

Gilligan, C. (1982). *In a different voice.* Cambridge, MA: Harvard University Press.

Goodheart, C.D. (1989). Short-term dynamic psychotherapy with difficult clients. In P.S. Keller and S.R. Heyman (Eds.), *Innovations in clinical practice: A source book* (pp. 15-26). Professional Resource Exchange: Sarasota, Florida.

Lazarus, R. (1982). Lectures presented at course *Stress and Coping.* Albert Einstein Summer Program, Cape Cod, MA.

Massie, M.J., Holland, J.C., & Straker, N. (1990). Psychotherapeutic interventions. In J.C. Holland & J.H. Rowland (Eds.), *Handbook of psychooncology* (pp. 455-469). New York: Oxford University Press.

Miller, J.B. (1976). *Toward a new psychology of women.* Boston: Beacon Press.

Ochberg, F.M. (1991, Spring) Post-traumatic therapy. *Psychotherapy, 28,*(1), 245-251.

Parad, H.J. (Ed.). (1965). *Crisis intervention: Selected readings.* New York: Family Service Association of America.

Puryear, D.A. (1979). *Helping people in crisis.* San Francisco: Jossey-Bass.

Schneidman, E.(1985). *Definition of suicide.* New York: John Wiley and Sons.

Tannen, D. (1990). *You just don't understand: Women and men in conversation.* New York: Wm. Morrow and Co.

Support Groups/ Group Therapy

Levine, B. (1979). *Group psychotherapy: Practice and development.* New Jersey: Prentice/Hall.

Lonergan, E.C. (1989). *Group intervention.* New Jersey: Aronson.

Moos, R. (1977). *Coping with physical illness.* New Jersey: Plenum.

Rutan, J.S. & Stone, W.N. (1984). *Psychodynamic group psychotherapy.* Massachusetts: D.C. Heath.

Spiegel, D., Bloom, J.R., Kraemer, H.C. & Gottheil, E. (1989). Effect of psychosocial treatment on survival of patients with metastatic breast cancer. *The Lancet, #8668,* pp. 888-891.

Spiegel, D., & Spira, J. (1991). *Supportive-expresive group therapy: A treatment manual of psychosocial intervention for women with recurrent breast cancer.* Psychosocial Treatment Laboratory, Stanford University School of Medicine.

Spira, J., & Spiegel, D. (1991). Group psychotherapy in the medically ill. In B. Fogel, & A. Stoudemire (Eds.), *Principles of medical psychiatry,* (2nd ed.) New York: American Psychiatric Press.

Yalom, Irwin. (1975). *The theory and practice of group psychotherapy.* New York: Basic Books.

Special Populations

American Association of Retired Persons. (1991). *Chances are...you need a mammogram.* (PF 4730). Bethesda, Maryland: Author.

American Cancer Society. (1986). *Breast reconstruction after mastectomy* (4630 PS Handout).

American Psychological Association. (1991). Bias in psychotherapy with lesbians and gay men. Report of task force on psychotherapy with lesbian and gay men. Washington, DC: Author.

Bray, S. & Siegal, D.L. (1987). Cancer. In P.B. Doress & D.L. Siegal (Eds.), *Ourselves growing older* (pp. 327-350). New York: Simon and Schuster.

Burg, M.A., Lane, D.S., & Polednak, A.P. (1990). Age group differences in the use of breast cancer screening tests. *Journal of Aging and Health, 2,* 514-530.

Chu, J., Diehr, P., Feigl, P., Glaefke, G., Begg,C., Glicksman, A. & Ford,L. (1987). The effect of age on the care of women with breast cancer in community hospital. *Journal of Gerontology, 42,* 185-190.

Fox, S.A. & Stein, J.A. (1991). The effect of physician-patient communication on mammography utilization by different ethnic groups. *Medical Care, 29,* 1065-1082.

Funch, D.P. (1987). Survival for breast and cervical cancer. In Stellman, S. (Ed.), *Women and cancer* (pp. 37-54). New York: Harrington Park Press.

Jarrett, J.R. (1988). Prophylactic mastectomy with immediate reconstruction. In Gant, T. & Vasconez, L. (Eds.), *Post mastectomy reconstruction* (pp. 125-149). Baltimore: Williams & Wilkins.

Kennedy, B.J. (1992). Aging and cancer. In Balducci, Erschler & Lyman, *Geriatric oncology* (pp3-7). Philadelphia: J.B. Lippincott.

Kennedy, B.J. (in press). Specific considerations for the older patient with cancer. In Calabresi & Schein (Eds.), *Medical oncology.* McGraw Hill. New York: NY.

Lashley, M.E. (1987). Predictors of breast self-examination practice among elderly women. *Advances in Nursing Science, 9,* 25-43.

Lourde, A. (1980). *The cancer journals.* San Francisco: Spinster/Aunt Lute.

National Cancer Institute. (1987). *Good news for blacks about cancer.* (NIH Publication No. 87-2956). Washington, DC: U.S. Government Printing Office.

National Cancer Institute. (1990). *Questions and answers about breast lumps.* (NIH Publication No. 90-2401). Washington, DC: U.S. Government Printing Office.

National Cancer Institute. (1990). *Smart advice for women 40 and over.* (NIH Publication No. 90-1581). Washington, DC: U.S. Government Printing Office.

National Cancer Institute. (1991). *Breast exams: What you should know.* (NIH Publication No. 91-2000). Washington, DC: U.S. Government Printing Office.

National Cancer Institute. (1992). *Breast cancer background.* (Fact Sheet 1196 FS). Washington, DC: U.S. Government Printing Office.

National Coalition for Cancer Survivorship. (1991) *Teamwork: The cancer patient's guide to talking with your doctor.* Silver Spring, MD: Author.

Newell, G.R. & Mills, P.K. (1987). Low cancer rates in Hispanic women related to social and economic factors. In Stellman, S. (Ed.), *Women and cancer* (pp. 23-35). New York: Harington Park Press.

Osborne, M.P. & Bayle, J.C. (1988). We would vary rarely recommend prophylactic mastectomy. *Primary Care & Cancer, 8,* 25-31.

Royak-Schaler, R. (1992). *Challenging the breast cancer legacy.* New York: Harper Collins.

Satariano, W.A., Ragheb, N.E., Buck, K.A., Swanson, G.M., & Branch, L.G. (1989). Aging and breast cancer: A case-control comparison of instrumental functioning. *Journal of Aging and Health, 1,* 209-233.

Zapka, J.G., Stoddard, A., Barth, R., Costanza, M.E., & Mas, E. (1989). Breast cancer screening utilization by Latina community health center clients. *Health Education Research Theory and Practice, 4,* 461-468.

Husbands and Significant Others

Lichtman, R. (1982). *Close relationships after breast cancer.* Unpublished doctoral dissertation, University of California, Los Angeles, California. In Northouse L., Cracchiolo-Caraway A., and Pappas-Appel, C. (1991) Psychologic consequences of breast cancer on partner and family. Seminars in Oncology Nursing 7, 216-223.

Lichtman, R., & Taylor, S. (1986). Close relationships and the female cancer patient. In Anderson B.L. (Ed.), *Women with cancer: Psychological perspectives.* (pp. 257-288). New York: Springer-Verlag.

Rowland, J.H., (1990).Interpersonal resources: Social support. In Holland and Rowland (Eds.), *Handbook of psychooncology* (pp. 58-71). New York: Oxford University Press.

Vinokur, A., & Vinokur-Kaplan, D. (1990). In sickness and in health: patterns of social support and undermining in older married couples. *Journal of Aging and Health, 2,* 215-241.

Helping the Children

American Cancer Society (1986). Helping children understand: A guide for a parent with cancer: (Handout).

Strauss, L.L. (1986). What about me? *A booklet for teenage children of cancer patients.* Cincinnati, Ohio: Cancer Family Care, Inc.

Thurber, J. (1990). *Many moons* (rev. ed.). New York: Harcourt, Brace, Jovanovich.

Specific Interventions

Cousins, N. (1989). *Head first.* New York: Penguin Books.

Edgar, E.N., Rosberger, Z. & Nowlis, D. (1992). Coping with cancer during the first year after diagnosis. *Cancer, 69,* (3).

Golden, W.L., Gersh, W., & Robbins, D.M. (1992). *Psychological treatment of cancer patients: A cognitive behavioral approach.* Boston: Allyn and Bacon.

Kubler-Ross, E. (1978). *On death and dying.* New York: Macmillan.

Lowen, A., & Lowen, L. (1977). *The way to vibrant health.* New York: Harper and Row.

Simonton, O.C., Mathew-Simonton, S., & Creighton, J.L. (1980). *Getting well again.* New York: Bantam Books.

Research On the Effectiveness of Psychological Interventions

Bartrop, R., Luckhurst, E., Lazarus, L., Kiloh, L., & Penny, R. (1977). Depressed lymphocyte function after bereavement. *Lancet, 1,* 834-836.

Benson, H. (1975). *The relaxation response.* New York: William Morrow & Company, Inc.

Blalock, J., Harbour-McMenamin, D., & Smith, E. (1985). Peptide hormones shared by the neuroendocrine and immunologic systems. *Journal of Immunology, 135,* 858-861.

Burish, T., Shartner, C., & Lyles, J. (1981). Effectiveness of multiple site EMG biofeedback and relaxation in reducing the aversiveness of cancer chemotherapy. *Biofeedback Self Regulation, 6,* 523-35.

Cangello, V. (1961). Hypnosis for the patient with cancer. *American Journal of Clinical Hypnosis, 4,* 215-226.

Clawson, T., & Swade R. (1975). The hypnotic control of blood flow and pain. *American Journal of Clinical Hypnosis, 17,* 160-69.

Dobkin, P., Zeichner, A., & Dickson-Parnell, B. (1985). Concomitants of anticipatory nausea and emesis in cancer chemotherapy. *Psychological Reports, 56,* 671-76.

Eysenck, H. & Grossarth-Maticek, R. (1991). Creative novation behaviour therapy as a prophylactic treatment for cancer and coronary heart disease, Part 2: Effects of treatment. *Behaviour Research & Therapy, 29,* 17-31.

Fawzy, F., Kemeny, M., Fawzy, N., Elashoff, R., Morton, D., Cousins, N., & Fahey, J. (1990). A structured psychiatric intervention for cancer patients, II: changes over time in immunological measures. *Archives of General Psychiatry, 47,* 729-735.

Grindler, J., & Bandler, R. (1981). *TRANCE-formations: neurolinguistic programming and the structure of hypnosis.* Utah: Real People Press.

Grossarth-Maticek, R., & Eysenck, H. (1989). Length of survival as a function of psychotherapy. *Psychological Reports, 65,* 315-21.

Kiecolt-Glaser, J., Fisher, L., Ogrocki, P., Stout, J., Speicher, C., & Glaser, R. (1987). Marital quality, marital disruption and immune function. *Psychosomatic Medicine, 49,* 13-34.

Kiecolt-Glaser, J., Glaser, R., Dyer, C., Shuttleworth, E., Ogrocki, P., & Speicher, C. (1987). Chronic stress and immunity in family caregivers of Alzheimer's disease victims. *Psychosomatic Medicine, 49,* 523-535.

Lea, P., Ware, P., & Monroe, R. (1960). The hypnotic control of intractable pain. *American Journal of Clinical Hypnosis, 3,* 3-8.

Levy, S., Herberman, R., Maluish, A., Schlien, B., & Lippman, M. (1985). Prognostic risk assessment in primary breast cancer by behaviorial and immuniligical parameters. *Health Psychology, 4,* 99-113.

Levy, S., Herberman, R., Whiteside, T., Sanzo, K., Lee, J., & Kirkwood, J. (1990). Perceived social support and tumor estrogen/progesterone receptor status as predictors of natural killer cell activity in breast cancer patients. *Psychosomatic Medicine, 52,* 73-85.

Levy, S., & Wise, B. (1988). Psychosocial risk factors and cancer progression. In C.L. Cooper (Ed.), *Stress and breast cancer,* New York: John Wiley & Sons Ltd.

Lyles, J., Burish, T., Krozely, M., & Oldham, R. (1982). Efficacy of relaxation training and guided imagery in reducing the aversiveness of cancer chemotherapy. *Journal of Consulting and Clinical Psychology, 50,* 509-524.

Massie, M.J., Holland, J.C., & Straker, N. (1990). Psychotherapeutic interventions. In J.C. Holland and J.H. Rowland (Eds.), *Handbook of psychooncology (pp. 455-469).* New York: Oxford University Press.

McKinnon, W., Weisse, C., Reynolds, C., Bowles, C., & Baum, A. (1989). Chronic stress, leucocyte subpopulations and humoral response to latent viruses. *Health Psychology, 8,* 389-402

Morganstern, H., Geilert, G., Walter, S., Ostfeld, A., & Siegel, B. (1984). The impact of a psychosocial support program on survival with breast cancer: the importance of selection bias in program evaluation. *Journal of Chronic Disease, 37,* 273-82.

Morrow, G., & Morrell, B. (1982). Behavioral treatment for the anticipatory nausea and vomiting induced by cancer chemotherapy. *New England Journal of Medicine, 307,* 1476-1480.

Pennebaker, J., Kiecolt-Glaser, J., & Glaser, R. (1988). Disclosure of traumas and immune function: health implications for psychotherapy. *Journal of Consulting and Clinical Psychology, 56,* 239-245.

Redd, W., Andresen, G., & Minagawa, R. (1982). Hypnotic control of anticipatory emesis in cancer patients receiving chemotherapy. *Journal of Consulting and Clinical Psychology, 50,* 14-19.

Spiegel, D. (1985). *The use of hypnosis in controlling cancer pain.* New York: American Cancer Society.

Spiegel, D., Bloom, J., Kraemer, H., & Gottheil, E. (1989). Effect of psychosocial treatment on survival of patients with metastatic breast cancer. *The Lancet, #8668,* pp. 888-891.

Waxler-Morrison, N., Hislop, T., Mears, B., & Kan, L. (1991). Effects of social relationships on survival for women with breast cancer: a prospective study. *Social Science and Medicine, 33,* 177-183.

Weisman, A., & Worden, J. (1975). Psychosocial analysis of cancer deaths. *Omega, 6,* 1075.

INDEX